MORE PRAISE FOR
THE REMEDY

"A welcome trend in clinical education and practice involves inviting patients and clients to tell their own stories of identity, illness, health care and resilience in their own words, to both learners and practitioners. *The Remedy* provides a rich tapestry of narratives across the spectrum of human sexuality and genders, and includes descriptions of innovations from committed health professionals who address the many gaps in providing attuned, informed care to queer and trans people."
—Allan Peterkin, MD, and co-author of
Caring for Lesbian and Gay People: A Clinical Guide

"*The Remedy* is a bandage lovingly placed on the open wounds of every LGBTQAI person afraid of going to a doctor. This book does not just ask doctors to follow the oath of "first do no harm"; it also demands medical practitioners respect, understand, and affirm our queer lives, bodies, and families. The Remedy is the collection of healing and solidarity queers desperately need."
—Sassafras Lowrey, author of *Lost Boi*

"*The Remedy* is a book to give to anyone working in health care, to queer and trans friends struggling to find their voice through an illness, to your straight parents and queer or trans children. The candour in this collection filled me with that relief and gratitude one senses from feeling deeply seen. Here are quintessential stories of queer and trans people navigating our health care and medical systems. If you're queer or trans, these confidences will be nothing short of healing.
If you're a medical practitioner, they'll be vital."
—Michael V. Smith, author of *My Body Is Yours*

"The best kind of waiting-room reading, *The Remedy* brings together many voices to offer something we often don't find through our health-care providers. Zena Sharman has collected points of view from many sides of medical interactions, creating a community of people who truly believe that the barriers to medical access that LGBTQIA people face are unjust but changeable."
—Rae Spoon, author of *First Spring Grass Fire*

THE REMEDY

QUEER AND TRANS VOICES
ON HEALTH AND HEALTH CARE

Edited by
ZENA SHARMAN

ARSENAL
PULP PRESS
VANCOUVER

SECOND PRINTING: 2017

ARSENAL PULP PRESS
Suite 202 – 211 East Georgia St.
Vancouver, BC V6A 1Z6
Canada
arsenalpulp.com

The publisher gratefully acknowledges the support of the Canada Council for the Arts and the British Columbia Arts Council for its publishing program, and the Government of Canada (through the Canada Book Fund) and the Government of British Columbia (through the Book Publishing Tax Credit Program) for its publishing activities.

 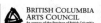 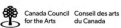 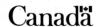

Design and cover illustration by Oliver McPartlin
Edited by Brian Lam with Linda Field
Editorial assistance by Claire Matthews
Illustrations for Innovation Profiles by Sam Bradd

Printed and bound in Canada

Library and Archives Canada Cataloguing in Publication:
    The remedy: queer and trans voices on health and health care / edited by Zena Sharman.

Includes bibliographical references.

Issued in print and electronic formats.

ISBN 978-1-55152-658-4 (paperback).—ISBN 978-1-55152-659-1

(html)

    1. Gays—Medical care. 2. Gays—Health and hygiene.
3. Transgender people--Medical care. 4. Transgender people—
Health and hygiene. I. Sharman, Zena, 1979-, editor

RA564.9.H65R44 2016   362.1086'64   C2016-904412-2
                                               C2016-904413-0

CONTENTS

INTRODUCTION

Why Queer and Trans Health Stories Matter

Zena Sharman

I'm at my friends' house for dinner, perched on a barstool in front of a kitchen island stocked with snacks. Four of us are gathered around the food, all queer, one trans. Two of my companions are cancer survivors who trade stories about treatments, symptoms, and chronic pain. They share a kinship and a form of solidarity that I'm grateful to witness. The rest of us listen intently as one describes a cross-border search and reading hundreds of plastic surgery journal articles in search of a cure for an injury they'd sustained during a botched diagnostic procedure, something doctors told them would inevitably lead to surgery and living the rest of their life with a colostomy bag. I hold my breath, tense with anticipation as my friend's tale of tenacity and self-advocacy unfolds, exhale a sigh of relief as they recount the final, triumphant chapter. It seems sweeter, queerer somehow that the story ends with a miracle cure in San Francisco.

I glance at my phone, a reflexive action I repeat casually and almost without thinking many times a day. This time, the words on the screen grab my full attention, fill me with a mix of empathy and rage as I read a text from a friend, upset and triggered following a violating encounter with a physician. She's a visibly queer Aboriginal person with a masculine gender presentation. This shouldn't be relevant to her traumatic medical experience, but it is, because mine probably would've been different. I'm a white femme with a PhD, prone to geeking out with my care providers about health research during appointments. No doctor has ever treated me the way they treated my friend. I sit with her words for a moment, take them in, feel acutely aware

9

of how my gender and white privilege shape the inequity of our experiences. I tell my friend how sorry I am that this happened to her, affirm that the doctor's behaviour was awful and inappropriate. I channel my anger into looking up information on how to file a complaint against a physician, send it to her, and hope that my friend's grievance is taken seriously, that there's some remedy, some recourse, that this doesn't happen to anybody else.

My hair stylist—a fellow queer femme—is cutting my hair and updating me about her efforts to get pregnant through IVF. She's being implanted with her partner's egg and donor sperm. They're paying out of pocket at the fertility clinic known as the go-to place for queers in Vancouver, but the rainbow flag on the website doesn't protect against the kind of institutionalized heteronormativity they encounter at every turn. I watch her in the mirror as she tells me about how the clinic keeps mixing her up with her partner when it communicates with them by phone or email, how they were given an information sheet for straight couples and told to "ignore the instructions for the man." I go on a feminist rant about patriarchy and evidence-based medicine when she describes how the clinic told her not to have an orgasm for three weeks after the first implantation attempt. Later, I post a question about the validity of these instructions on social media. A group of mostly queer friends that includes a midwife, a labour and delivery nurse, a naturopath, several of North America's leading sex researchers, and a handful of parents collectively arrive at an answer. They don't make pamphlets for this sort of thing.

A common thread connects these narratives: the power of stories and how health information circulates in queer and trans communities. Who the good queer- and trans-competent family doctors are (and who's accepting patients). How to navigate the process of getting public funding for gender-affirming surgery and how to heal from that surgery—all of the things not captured in the surgeon's standard post-operative instruction sheet—like my friends the cancer survivors, the kind of knowledge you only accumulate by living it.

How to find a queer- and trans-savvy trauma-informed therapist who won't pathologize your sexual or relational choices and who isn't dating your closest friend or your ex or both, and who ideally has a sliding scale. Who makes the best unscented styling products so you can be an ally to your friends with chemical sensitivities *and* have awesome hair. Which STI clinic has the cool tattooed nurses who don't bat an eye at what you did last weekend and who bring respect, knowledge, and empathy into every encounter.

And horror stories, too: health care providers and clinics to avoid. Asking for support and validation from friends after being repeatedly referred to by the wrong name or the wrong gender pronoun during a health care visit. Dealing with the physical, emotional, and economic implications of being unable to find or access or afford the essential health services you so desperately need. Crowdfunding campaigns urgently seeking to fill the places where the system or the social safety net falls short. Memorial after memorial after memorial for friends and loved ones lost to violence or suicide. Our community is no stranger to loss, to individual and collective trauma, to lives lived in the gaps and the in-between places.

We make do and we re-make. We crowdsource our health in a community with a long history of caring for one another outside of and often in spite of dominant systems and structures. We document and gather and share information, filling the gaps in the evidence where our lives, needs, and identities are increasingly but still insufficiently visible. We tell stories, and we take care of each other.

There's a rich and growing literature on queer and trans health, but it seems to me that people's stories are missing from a conversation that's often centred on things like research data and guidelines for health care providers. *The Remedy* puts queer and trans voices at the centre of this conversation. I can trace the origins of this anthology back to "sexual medicine day," when I spent an afternoon in a classroom full of first-year medical students. Several hundred of them listened intently as my colleagues and I delivered an introductory lecture on queer and trans health. We talked about terminology, disparities, stigma, and resilience, gave tips on inclusive and affirming care. After class I joined in on one of the tutorials where I answered students' questions about my queer life and identity. Their desire to become competent, respectful clinicians was palpable, as was their appetite for information. I felt acutely aware of the power of connection in that moment, of what can happen when we pair research evidence and clinical guidelines with people's stories. Of how powerful it can be to just sit down together and talk to each other.

It's no wonder those first-year medical students were hungry for knowledge. They're learning in an environment where relatively little time is dedicated to formal training on queer and trans health. A recent survey of 150 Canadian and US medical schools reported a median of five hours dedicated to teaching this content in the entire curriculum, and about 40 percent of institutions rated their curricular content as only "fair" in quality.[1] Consider this in the context of US data from a survey of 4,400 straight first-year medical students.[2] The study found that 46 percent of them expressed at least some explicit (conscious) bias against gay and lesbian people, and 82 percent held at least some degree of implicit (unconscious) bias against them. The study also found that more frequent and more positive intergroup contact between these students and sexual minorities predicted more positive attitudes toward them.

1 Juno Obedin-Maliver, et al., "Lesbian, Gay, Bisexual, and Transgender–Related Content in Undergraduate Medical Education," *Journal of the American Medical Association* 306 (9) (2011): 971-77.

2 S.E. Burke, et al., "Do Contact and Empathy Mitigate Bias Against Gay and Lesbian People Among Heterosexual First-Year Medical Students? A Report From the Medical Student CHANGE Study," *Academic Medicine* 90 (5) (May 2015): 645-51.

I don't mean to single out medical students or doctors. The entire health care system is implicated in creating a "persistent, negative culture ... toward sexual and gender minority populations" that manifests as stigma and discrimination and exerts a powerful influence on health disparities.[3]

A 2010 Lambda Legal survey on health care discrimination found that 56 percent of lesbian, gay or bisexual respondents, 70 percent of trans and gender non-conforming respondents, and almost 63 percent of people living with HIV had experienced at least one of the following types of discrimination: being refused needed care; health care providers refusing to touch them or using excessive precautions; providers using harsh or abusive language; being blamed for their health status; providers being physically rough or abusive.[4] In almost every category of this survey, trans and gender non-conforming people reported the highest rates of discrimination and barriers to care, and a higher proportion of respondents who were people of colour or low-income reported experiencing discriminatory and substandard care. Most of the people who participated in this survey expected to experience discrimination from their health care providers.

Let me say that again: *most of the people who participated in this survey expected to experience discrimination from their health care providers.*

For those of you who are shocked or angered by this revelation: I want you to sit with this feeling for a moment. Feel it in your body. Hold it in your heart. Use it as part of the foundation for your allyship, for the active and embodied work of solidarity.

Now keep reading.

3 M. Mansh G. Garcia, M.R. Lunn, "From patients to providers: changing the culture in medicine toward sexual and gender minorities," *Academic Medicine* 90 (5) (May 2015): 574-80.

4 Lambda Legal, *When Health Care Isn't Caring: Lambda Legal's Survey on Discrimination Against LGBT People and People Living with HIV* (2010), http://www.lambdalegal.org/sites/default/files/publications/downloads/whcic-report_when-health-care-isnt-caring.pdf

And then there are those of you who are thinking, "Tell me something I didn't already know," because you've become so accustomed to weighing the likelihood of discrimination or mistreatment by your health care providers against the severity of your health concerns. That's assuming you have access to health care in the first place, something many folks struggle with for a whole host of reasons.

To you, I offer this apology: I am so sorry that the system is failing you, that your health care providers are failing you, that we are failing you. You deserve so much better.

It doesn't take a PhD or a medical degree to figure out that experiencing systemic discrimination is lousy for your health. It's as intuitive as it is complex. Whole books have been written about queer and trans health disparities and how to resolve them through research and care—here I'm thinking of landmark texts like the Institute of Medicine's *The Health of Lesbian, Gay, Bisexual, and Transgender People* (2011), *Trans Bodies, Trans Selves* (2014), and *The Fenway Guide to Lesbian, Gay, Bisexual, and Transgender Health, 2nd Edition* (2015). These books are beside me on the kitchen table as I write these words. I keep them near me for reference and inspiration. I feel grateful to their authors, grateful that these books exist, grateful for the weight of their authority in a world that often feels like it's trying to disappear us, tell us that our concerns don't matter, that we shouldn't be so sensitive, that it's our fault, that we should do as we're told, take what we're offered, say thank you, shut up.

I feel the weight of this awareness as I face the overwhelming prospect of trying to summarize the complexities of queer and trans health in a paragraph or two. There's no monolithic experience, no simple narrative, no easy way to lump and slice the incredible diversity that characterizes queer and trans identities, communities, and lives. Even my terminology is inadequate— "queer" and "trans" are imperfect shorthand for sexual orientations and gender identities including and certainly not limited to lesbian, gay, bisexual, queer, asexual, pansexual, Two-Spirit, transgender, transsexual, intersex, and so many more. And these identities don't exist in isolation. Black feminist scholar Kimberlé Williams Crenshaw[5] was the first to describe this in terms of intersectionality—that is, how gender and sexuality intersect with race, ethnicity, indigeneity, ability, body size, age, class, income, education, place, and other facets of identity and experience. Privilege and oppression intersect with and derive from homophobia, biphobia, transphobia, racism, colonialism, ableism, fatphobia, sexism, classism, ageism, and so on; they are as present in and shaping of whole systems of care as they are in individual lives.

You need to understand this context in order to understand why trans folks tend to fare worse than cisgender folks, and why trans women experience the health impacts of transmisogyny. Why queer and trans people of colour and Indigenous people experience poorer health outcomes than their white peers. Why poor and working-class queers have greater health disparities than wealthy ones. Why borders, geography, and where you live have an enormous influence on your access to health care. Why all of this is a result of health being rooted in complex structures of privilege and oppression, not because being queer or trans is inherently bad for your health.

If you're still hungry for statistics—numbers to prove what many of us already know in our bodies, our blood, our bones, our hearts, our spirits, our memories—I encourage you to read the appendix to this introduction. I'm a researcher by training, I understand why facts and percentages and citations feel concrete and understandable. Comforting, even. Something to hold onto. This book isn't about statistics, though, and it's not about comfort. Some of the stories in *The Remedy* might make you uncomfortable. They might hit

5 Kimberlé Williams Crenshaw, "Mapping the Margins: Intersectionality, Identity Politics, and Violence against Women of Color," *Stanford Law Review* 43 (6) (1991):1241-99.

too close to home, might trigger a memory of an awful health care encounter or a time you really screwed up with a client or patient or friend. They might make you realize that you're screwing up right now. Many of these stories bear witness to the lived experiences of systemic and individual failures of care.

But *The Remedy* is also about hope and resilience—an affirmation that we are here, that we are amazingly strong, that we deserve more, that people and providers and systems can do so much better, and that in many contexts, they already are. More than thirty people from across North America share their experiences in this collection, each essay or poem or drawing a testament to the lifesaving necessity of queer and trans stories. These stories are interspersed with short profiles on a handful of innovative queer and trans health programs and projects, my effort to highlight some of the outstanding work being done by and with queer and trans communities. I hope it inspires more.

There's a great deal of honesty, courage, and vulnerability in these pages, people bravely sharing the truth of their lives as patients and health care providers, healers and students, activists and artists. This book grew out of my desire to see these stories, these voices, reflected on the page. I hope you recognize parts of yourself in this book, that it makes you ask questions, teaches you something. I hope it makes you happy and sad and angry, that you notice all of the things that are missing from it. *The Remedy* isn't the whole story of queer and trans health; it's part of an ongoing conversation. I hope you add your voice and your story to it, too. May we all listen and bear witness to one another, and may we all join together in the fight for queer and trans health.

APPENDIX

An Incomplete and Highly Oversimplified Summary of Some of What
We Know About Queer and Trans Health Disparities

I thought long and hard about whether or not to include this appendix in *The Remedy*. It's impossible to reduce the diversity and complexity of queer and trans health, identities, and lives into a single statistic. I'm not attempting to be comprehensive—rather, I'm aiming to present some of what we know about queer and trans health disparities as a way to help those of you who are less familiar with them understand the health impacts of homophobia, transphobia, and biphobia.

As you read, I urge you to put this information in context: think about the social determinants of health, about stigma, discrimination, and structural violence, and about intersectionality. Understand how racism and colonialism exacerbate the effects of these disparities for queer and trans people who are Indigenous or people of colour. Appreciate that research is a helpful tool while remembering that many people's identities, lives, and stories are still missing from the data, for all kinds of reasons. Remember the histories of those who came before us, and endeavour to respect and learn from these legacies while working to shape the future. Know in your mind, your heart, and your bones how magnificently resilient queer and trans people and communities are. Keep learning, keep listening, keep reading, keep asking questions about queer and trans health and why these disparities persist. Above all, keep working for change. This story is still being told.

A note on terminology: while I've intentionally used the more general language of "queer and trans" throughout my contributions to this collection, the information presented below reflects the language used in the original source.

Health care utilization and access to care

+ One in five transgender people report having been denied care by a doctor. Trans people of colour are even more likely to report being denied care.[1]

+ Transgender people are more likely than cisgender people to be uninsured. They're also more likely to postpone medical care because of being uninsured and because of experiences with discrimination.[2]

+ Nearly half of trans women and men in a Canadian study reported feeling uncomfortable discussing trans health issues with their family doctors, and almost 40 percent of them reported at least one trans-specific negative experience with their doctors.[3]

+ The same study showed that over half of the trans participants who'd accessed care through hospital emergency departments (ED) reported trans-specific negative experiences. One-fifth of them reported avoiding ED care because they were concerned their trans status would negatively affect their experience.[4]

+ Lesbians and bisexual women may use preventive health services less often than heterosexual women.[5]

+ Lesbian, gay, bisexual, and transgender elders may experience additional barriers to accessing care due to a lack of culturally appropriate social services and providers.[6]

Stigma, discrimination, violence, and trauma

+ Lesbian, gay, bisexual, and transgender people frequently experience stigma, discrimination, and violence because of their sexual- and gender-minority status.[7]

+ Compared to straight people, lesbian, gay, and bisexual people have double the risk of exposure to traumatic experiences over their lifetimes.[8]

+ Lesbian, gay, bisexual, and transgender people are at higher lifetime risk of violent victimization and maltreatment than straight, cisgender people.[9]

+ Twenty percent of participants in a Canadian trans health study reported having been the targets of physical or sexual assaults and another 34 percent had experienced verbal harassment or threats because of being trans.[10]

- Lesbian, gay, bisexual, and transgender youth report higher levels of violence, victimization, and harassment than their heterosexual and cisgender peers.[11]

- Lesbian, gay, bisexual, and transgender youth are more likely to be homeless. Many of those who access housing through the shelter system report experiencing homophobia, biphobia, and transphobia in that environment.[12]

Substance use

- Lesbian, gay, bisexual, and transgender populations have higher rates of tobacco, alcohol, and drug use than heterosexuals.[13]

- Lesbian, gay, bisexual, and transgender youth are more likely than their straight counterparts to use tobacco, alcohol, and drugs.[14]

- Bisexuals have twice the risk of smoking than heterosexuals.[15]

Mental health

- Lesbian, gay, bisexual, and transgender populations have higher rates of certain mental health issues.[16] For example, lesbian, gay, and bisexual adults seem to experience more mood and anxiety disorders and depression than heterosexual adults. They're also at higher risk for suicidal ideation and attempts.[17]

- A Canadian study found that about three-quarters of trans adults had ever seriously considered suicide and 43 percent had attempted suicide at some point in their lives. The same study showed that trans youth (up to age twenty-four) were nearly twice as likely to seriously consider suicide as those over the age of twenty-five, and almost three times as likely to have attempted suicide within the past year.[18]

- Lesbian, gay, and bisexual youth are twice as likely as their straight peers to have suicidal ideation, and they're four times as likely to make suicide attempts that require medical attention.[19]

Sexual health

- Gay and bisexual men (and other men who have sex with men) have higher rates of HIV and sexually transmitted infections (STIs). The prevalence of

19

these is higher for men of colour.[20]

+ Studies have shown higher rates of HIV-related risk factors and HIV/AIDS among gay, lesbian, bisexual, transgender and Two-Spirit Aboriginal people in Canada.[21]

+ Trans women have higher rates of HIV and STIs, particularly trans women of colour.[22]

+ Experiences of racism and transphobia have been shown to interact to increase HIV risk among Aboriginal and trans people of colour.[23]

Cancer and chronic disease

+ Gay men are at higher risk of anal cancer than straight men.[24]

+ Lesbians and bisexual women tend to have higher rates of breast cancer, and are less likely to get preventive services for cancer.[25]

+ There's little data on cancer prevalence or outcomes for trans and gender nonconforming populations, signaling a need for more research in this area.[26]

+ Lesbian, gay and bisexual adults have 1.5 times the risk of asthma compared to heterosexuals.[27]

+ When compared with straight men, young gay and bisexual men tend to show significant elevations in the biomarkers of cardiovascular disease.[28]

1 AAMC's Advisory Committee on Sexual Orientation, Gender Identity, and Sex Development, *Implementing Curricular and Institutional Climate Changes to Improve Health Care for Individuals Who are LGBT, Gender Nonconforming, or Born with DSD: A Resource for Medical Educators* (Washington: Association of American Medical Colleges, 2014).

2 Ibid.

3 G.R. Bauer, et al., "Factors Impacting Transgender Patients' Discomfort with their Family physicians: A Respondent Driven Sampling Study," *PLoS ONE* 10, no. 12 (2015): e0145046.

4 G.R. Bauer, et al., "Reported Emergency Department Avoidance, Use, and Experiences of Transgender Persons in Ontario, Canada: Results from a Respondent-Driven Sampling Survey," *Annals of Emergency Medicine* 63, no. 6 (2014): 713-20.

5 Committee on Lesbian, Gay, Bisexual, and Transgender Health Issues and Research Gaps and Opportunities, *The Health of Lesbian, Gay, Bisexual, and Transgender People: Building a Foundation for Better Understanding* (Washington: Institute of Medicine, The National Academies Press, 2011).

6 H.J. Makadon, et al., *Fenway Guide to Lesbian, Gay, Bisexual, and Transgender Health, 2nd Ed.* (Philadelphia: American College of Physicians, 2015).

7 Committee on Lesbian, Gay, Bisexual, and Transgender Health Issues and Research Gaps and Opportunities, 2011.

8 AAMC, 2014.

9 Ibid.

10 K. Scanlon, et al., "Ontario's Trans Communities and Suicide: Transphobia is Bad for our Health," *Trans PULSE e-Bulletin*, 1 (2) (November 12, 2010). http://transpulseproject.ca/wp-content/uploads/2010/11/E2English.pdf

11 Committee on Lesbian, Gay, Bisexual, and Transgender Health Issues and Research Gaps and Opportunities, 2011.

12 The Homeless Hub. Lesbian, Gay, Bisexual, Transgender, Transsexual, Queer, Questioning and 2-Spirited (LGBTQ2) (2016). http://homelesshub.ca/about-homelessness/population-specific/lesbian-gay-bisexual-transgender-transsexual-queer

13 Makadon, et al., 2015.

14 Committee on Lesbian, Gay, Bisexual, and Transgender Health Issues and Research Gaps and Opportunities, 2011; AAMC, 2014.

15 AAMC, 2014.

16 Makadon, et al., 2015.

17 Committee on Lesbian, Gay, Bisexual, and Transgender Health Issues and Research Gaps and Opportunities, 2011.

18 Scanlon, et al., 2010.

19 Makadon, et al., 2015.

20 Ibid.

21 Public Health Agency of Canada, *Chapter 8: HIV/AIDS Among Aboriginal People in Canada (2014)*. http://www.phac-aspc.gc.ca/aids-sida/publication/epi/2010/8-eng.php

22 AAMC, 2014; Makadon et al., 2015.

23 R.K. Marcellin, et al, "Intersecting Impacts of Transphobia and Racism on HIV Risk Among Trans Persons of Colour in Ontario, Canada," *Ethnicity and Inequalities in Health and Social Care* 6, no. 4 (2013): 97-107.

24 AAMC, 2014.

25 Committee on Lesbian, Gay, Bisexual, and Transgender Health Issues and Research Gaps and Opportunities, 2011; Makadon et al, 2015.

26 E.T. Taylor and M.K. Bryson, "Cancer's Margins: Trans* and Gender Nonconforming People's Access to Knowledge, Experiences of Cancer Health, and Decision-Making," *LGBT Health* 3, no. 1 (2016): 79–89.

27 AAMC, 2014.

28 Ibid.

call in sick

Vivek Shraya

how many mornings
> don't
> count

how many mornings
> fresh slate sun rays hope
> eclipsed by reminder of your own body

how many mornings
> does it storm without storming
> do you feel eaten but don't feel like eating

how many mornings
> log in refresh dodge comments
> scan comments log out restart

how many mornings
> tally likes for love wonder what a click tap
> from a stranger grants you that you can't grant
> yourself what the lack of a click tap takes
> from you that you can't give yourself

how many mornings
> google *toronto tallest bridges subway suicides*
> "only 60 percent who jump die"

how many mornings
> *you have run out of sick days*
> when do you run out of being brown?

Trans folks are often expected to embrace a narrative that makes cis people comfortable—something simple and linear that upholds their binary understanding of gender transition. Whether that means denying our current identities or our past ones, it's a saddening distraction to once again have to contort myself so that my service provider is comfortable enough to work with me.

NAME GAME

Being Seen In My Entirety

Kyle Shaughnessy

Using my new name and pronouns for the first time was a pretty nerve-wracking experience. I didn't feel like I was finally being seen as the "real" me or like I was putting on a comfortable old sweater. It was very uncomfortable. The first time anyone called me Kyle and most definitely the first times anyone called me "he," I was mortified. All of a sudden I felt as if my gender issues were visible to the entire room. Like no one could use my new pronouns without seeing an image of me as a teenager contorting myself in baggy t-shirts in front of the mirror trying to flatten my chest. I felt like a joke. But I knew that in the long run it was what I wanted, so I trusted that all new things feel uncomfortable at first, even the good ones, and stuck with it. Now it feels like my name. A nice, one-syllable, age-appropriate name that contains all the letters of my birth name. It feels good when people use it, even if it's the only name they know. It feels like a signifier of respect. It *is* a signifier of respect. Although it seems very simple, having someone treat me as who I say I am (regardless of my driver's license or birth certificate) tells me that I will be safe enough accessing their services and support. This is particularly true when accessing medical and counselling services.

I dedicate a lot of time to working on myself. I love therapy. I think every adult who is privileged enough to have the means to access therapy should access it however they can, and I access it regularly. However, it's not easy to find a provider who has both a strong therapeutic skillset and gets the nuances (and not-so nuances) that go into doing effective work with trans folks. It's also quite common for service providers to write trans clients out of their practice altogether because of an assumption that we're a highly complex population that they wouldn't even know where to begin with. This is an excuse. Once you have a decent understanding of the systemic barriers we face and can comfortably employ concepts of basic respect for our identities, your other skills are still very handy. A trans person's panic attack can be remedied similarly to a cis person's panic attack—it just might be triggered by something different, like being misgendered.

Although I've had my share of less than stellar trans-friendly therapy, I've also had some pretty great experiences—specifically with a therapist I've known since just before my transition. Taking on the recent personal work of unpacking childhood trauma, I put the necessary trust in her when she asked how I'd like my past and present names and pronouns used. I became willing to take a risk because she thought to ask me, very comfortably and confidently, as though she asks this of everyone, "What can Kyle tell little Katie in there to help her feel safe when these memories surface? He is an adult now, a grown man who is no longer powerless in his life." She sees me in my entirety. She remembers my preference for being referred to by the relevant names at the appropriate times. There may be many trans folks for whom this doesn't work, even in regression therapy, as they might feel that their identity is being undermined or they aren't truly being respected for who they are. But it works for me.

My therapist is not queer, she is not trans, she is not really all that involved in the community, and does not go out of her way to name herself as an ally. She is simply very skilled at making people comfortable enough to do the healing they need to do. If I had told her that my self-concept involves being seen as a boy at age four, I know this would be honoured as well.

In the past, I've had service providers who know I'm trans (and have been given the same permission to use age-corresponding names/pronouns) refer to me as having been a little boy. This is distracting and takes me right out of the therapeutic moment. I didn't experience my childhood as a little boy, I experienced it as an adopted, half-breed reincarnation of Shirley Temple. I also didn't have the experience of being a tomboy—getting in fights, hunting for frogs, or playing street hockey. As far as I remember, I was perfectly happy being dressed up like a dolly. I also expected to become a flamboyant, artistic, and clever gay man when I grew up. And, having been relatively unaware of the rigid binary world of gender roles and expressions, I had absolutely no concept of anything being in the way of this. As a teenager I became a lot more of a tomboy—driving dangerously in crappy cars, listening to loud punk music, drinking hard liquor, and ~~riding~~ owning a skateboard. Still, I lived those years as a problematically angsty teenage girl.

So when a therapist refers to me as a "little Kyle" or "when you were a young boy," it tells me that coddling their own discomfort with my evolving gender identity is higher on their priority list than creating an effective therapeutic experience. It also tells me that they're distracted with trying to wrap their minds around my anatomy. This is disappointing and infuriating all at once, that the grip of the gender binary is tight enough to throw off someone who spends hours each week hearing people's innermost details. I'm not asking for anything all that complicated, really, even from service providers who've only completed a few hours of training on providing respectful care to trans folks.

Although familiarity with the technical aspects of gender transition is important, it is equally important to be able to welcome us in, on our own terms. Often, we have to leave parts of who we are at the door in order to receive the care we need. Ignoring who we were or dismissing who we now are prevents us from fully engaging in our own wellness. Trans folks are often expected to embrace a narrative that makes cis people comfortable—something simple and linear that upholds their binary understanding of gender transition. Whether that means denying our current identities or our past ones, it's a saddening distraction to once again have to contort myself so that my service provider is comfortable enough to work with me.

Nothing gets you more familiar and comfortable with the flux and fluidity of gender than working with trans, gender nonconforming, non-binary identified, and queer youth. As someone who has worked with trans youth for many years, I often explain to other service providers that while the constantly evolving language and concepts of gender and sexual identity in youth populations can be overwhelming at times, if we don't keep up we lose the ability to connect and therefore to do effective work. When we sign up as health care providers, educators, parents, we sign up to sometimes make ourselves uncomfortable in order to make our young people more comfortable.

I've met a lot of parents of trans and gender nonconforming youth; parents who know their child as Alysha (she), but who I also know as Aiden (he) at youth group and AJ (no pronouns) on social media. Due to a general lack of agency in their own lives, many trans and gender nonconforming youth are required to live with multiple identities. Their housing, food, employment, education, and other basic needs may be at the mercy of however comfortable their adult support systems are with these young people's gender identities. When I decided to become a youth worker I committed to putting young people's safety, comfort, and sense of belonging at the epicentre of my interactions with them. I make it a priority to learn which names and pronouns youth want or need used at which times, in which environments, in front of which people. I use them accordingly and understand the possible risks involved in making a mistake. This is the dance I signed up to do, and this is the dance my therapist is doing with me in her thoughtful, consensual, and respectful use of my names and pronouns.

Being able to effortlessly flow between pronouns, names, and identities in conversation—being able to weave these together in a way that fully honours and respects the person in front of you, however that looks for them, is a necessary skill. Whether you're going back and forth between versions of the person while speaking to them directly or whether you're keeping track of which version of them exists in which environment for their personal safety, it basically comes down to this: if you want to strengthen your relationship with your trans clients—respect us as who we say we are (and who we say we were), regardless of how we look, how we act, how you remember us, or who you expected us to become. Ask us who we are, how we want our histories to be honoured, and what respect looks like to us. You only get better at it with practice, genuine care, and humility.

The medical-industrial complex leaves trans and gender variant bodies yearning for attendance to needs long ignored. We are liminal. We are elusive. We live and breathe in defiance of a school of thought based on two genders, eternally rooted in two unchanging bodies.

UNLEARNING

improving trans care by reorienting medical and nursing discourse

soma navidson

This morning, members of my cohort and I met in the nursing skills lab to learn "code blue" skills on a mannequin. One of our group members said, "When they present us a scenario with a chick patient, why don't they make the mannequin a chick? It's so ... disorienting." This is only a tiny shard of the transphobic microaggressions which daily weigh on my chest, forcing all possible relief from my lungs. Every day in this cohort is a struggle, a fight for space to learn in a field that largely refuses to acknowledge that my body—and others like it—exists, let alone works to create an environment conducive to trans care.

I feel this struggle in my stomach, hot and nauseating. I imagine activating my liver. Livers filter toxins from the blood, break down old cells. In essence, they help bodies process and recycle. As it filters the poison, metabolizes the hurt, I reengage the situation. I learn how to respond to a cardiac event. While other people in the room get to call the end of the code, I leave in a state of emergency.

My first degree is in gender and women's studies and while I can talk about structures of (re)creation of gender and normativity all day long, I'm in nursing school so I know how to prioritize interventions: airway first. I've been taught both by my activism and now by my discipline to work from the most urgent and vulnerable to the least. Let's make some room to breathe before setting the rest of the system(s) in order. I exist. Other trans and genderqueer people exist. Some of us change our bodies, some do not; this is not dependent on categorical identification but personal preference and access to care.

Now that we're breathing, however shallow, let's turn our shovels around and dig upwards for a change, because we've been piling on the dirt of dominant discourse for a long time now. Nursing diagnoses tend to focus less on diagnostic evaluations of disease processes and more on how to negotiate bodily changes, social outcomes, and to reduce risk. Similarly, solutions to ciscentric health care provision must acknowledge the larger interlocking systems, get at the problem's root(s), and be as simple as possible.

The medical-industrial complex leaves trans and gender variant bodies yearning for attendance to needs long ignored. We are liminal. We are elusive. We live and breathe in defiance of a school of thought based on two genders, eternally rooted in two unchanging bodies. Still, individual providers and medical thought writ large consistently harm us emotionally, physically, spiritually. Trans and gender variant people are murdered, incarcerated, unemployed, homeless, commit suicide, are exposed to sexual violence and to HIV at rates higher than population average—this is especially true for trans women of colour.[1]

This is too toxic for my liver to break down. Cirrhosis. While ciscentric health care isn't solely responsible for any of this, it offers a broad-strokes

1 Pooja Gehi, "Struggles from the Margins: Anti-Immigrant Legislation and the Impact on Low-Income Transgender People of Color," *Women's Rights Law Report 30*, no. 2 (Winter 2009): 315-29; Trans Student Educational Resources, "Why Trans People Need More Visibility." Accessed June 30, 2015. http://www.transstudent.org/transvisibility

image of the scale of our marginalization. Trans and gender nonconforming people don't get care that we need because of systemic barriers, (conscious or unconscious) personal animosities, and often simply because no one has bothered to derive or provide such care.

For almost everyone in my cohort, including my professors, I'm the first (visibly) trans person they've met. Our needs, if they're discussed at all, are lumped in with larger "LGBT" needs; this is to say, they're basically not mentioned. Meanwhile, we're disregarded and disrespected on a daily basis. But each affront offers an opportunity to restructure how we think and talk about bodies, hopefully in ways that organically lead to higher quality trans care.

I'm in a physiology lecture. We're learning about the liver. Apparently it is "designed to process and filter blood." In this moment I realize a need to cultivate a practice of simultaneously unlearning while learning. Obviously I need to make grades and there's some really important knowledge that will enable me to become an effective care provider. Moreover, bodies are weird and gorgeous and I want to learn as much as I possibly can!

However, livers, like people, aren't "designed" to do anything; livers, like people, merely exist in relationship with what's around them. Unlike livers, which function in more mechanical ways, people are social creatures who shift and recreate themselves. Humans have agency. "Design" is a dangerous concept with strong implications that life was intentionally created, undermining our agency over our bodies and social roles. I don't accept "design," so I imagine new ways of understanding what is taught. Rather than "livers are designed to ..." my notes state "livers do ..."

Taste buds burn off my tongue as I bite back lightning bolts. They're bitter, acidotic like enzymes erupting from the base of my teeth to digest simple sugars. Fumes travel upward sending vapour toward my decidedly flared nostrils. My professor, as has often been the case in my nursing program, doesn't notice the rage pouring over my front row desk and billowing toward her like smog. She repeats herself: "There are three risk factors that you can never change: age, race, and gender. Don't forget them: age, race, and gender." While I know that race is also socially constructed and mishandled by the medical-industrial complex, my very breath proves the claim about gender brazenly incorrect.

I cannot count the number of times that my professors have referred to gender as "a non-modifiable risk factor."[2] They seem to have ignored my painful twinging every time it is expressed. This implies a link between gender and bodies while simultaneously denying the existence of trans people who are capable of and choose to alter our bodies medically. It's uncertain whether or not this belief changes our risk factors for things like congestive heart disease, because the research that claims gendered differences in risk doesn't include us. The research is based on cis men and cis women. It's unclear whether or not this has to do with hormone balances (or when in life these levels shift), cultural behavioral differences, or some other factor(s).

By focusing so recklessly on socially engrained ideas of gender, we enable the whole medical field to continue refusing to do research that is relevant to trans and gender variant people. This leaves us without knowledge upon which to base understandings of bodies that might, in some instances, require importantly different care. The care is then left to the behest of providers who are guessing at best, disproportionately exposing us to illness, poor health care, and death. This is oppression, but it is not without opportunity.

Instead this scenario could become a moment to discuss the interplay between research and health disparities. Or, until the right research exists, it could be a time to teach care providers the skills necessary to seek related

2 While some gender studies enthusiasts and would-be allies would see "gender" replaced with "sex," similar problems follow. The implication is that we have power over our genders but that our bodies are somehow inherently "sexed," leaving us disenfranchised in the hands of providers who think we're "male-bodied women" or "female-bodied men."

research to ensure their best guesses are better than they otherwise would have been. This is a moment to break down old and useless blood cells, to purge them from our body of medical knowledge. It's time to unlearn.

A guest lecturer in my pharmacology class mentions triamterene, a potassium-sparing diuretic.[3] I ask if it has similar anti-androgen properties to spironolactone. The people sitting around me don't know what this means and the lecturer doesn't have an answer. They all think that I'm inexplicably brilliant. I'm not. When my body was still producing testosterone, I took spironolactone to block its effects at the cellular level, making my skin softer, my body hair finer, etc. My knowledge came through personal experience.

Unlike livers, curriculum is designed. As people we have a marvelous capacity to respond to what's around us in intentional ways. Were our curriculum designed to address even the most surface levels of trans medical care, this wouldn't have been an unexpected or unanswerable question. It could have even helped us become more adept at medication provision. There are so many moments when trans and gender variant care could be explored, yet it is blatantly disregarded. Rather than building a separate trans curriculum, it makes more sense to incorporate trans concerns into all moments of our curriculum, because we're trans in all moments of accessing care, not just when accessing trans-specific care.

One sign of liver toxicity is chronic fatigue. Experiencing transphobic microaggressions daily is grueling. Like livers, I have a threshold. I exploded in class when my professor introduced genograms as a way to model families. "Family" is not a useful term in attempting to assess genetic risk for my queer self, as it's broad and amorphous. Family shifts and changes, with relationships often being based on anything but blood. Beyond the very uselessness of this technique for me and many others, the genogram samples provided are all

3 Triamterene and spironolactone are both potassium-sparing diuretics, but triamterene does not have anti-androgenic properties and spironolactone does.

based on two genders. A shape depicting one of two reductive genders must represent each family member. I wish I had been this articulate. Instead, I simply roar that most people in my family can't be represented this way, that this is violence, this is silencing.

I leave school gasping and crying. I'm terrified about what it may mean to be out at school. While I was almost certainly always out as trans, as it's consistently mapped onto my body by cissexist standards, I wasn't planning on hoisting a non-binary flag during week two. Sometimes, though, my rage and grief at the forces that render me and some of my deepest loves impossible gets the better of me. Sometimes my heart and my teeth become the same organ, biting for the sake of pumping blood. This shouldn't be my fight.

This shouldn't be anyone's fight. How hard, really, would it be to offer a genogram example with myriad gender possibilities—one that prioritizes the relationships that will be alongside an individual during her negotiation of health and illness as much or more than genetic risk factors? We can recast this to make space for people with diverse relationship structures and genders. Creating a template for our existence within nursing and medical discourse would help providers learn to validate our lived experiences and in turn provide more holistic care.

We're learning about benign prostatic hypertrophy. My professor bluntly states, "Every male is going to experience some kind of benign prostatic hypertrophy if they live long enough." I find my mind wandering, wondering about my own prostate. I had surgery a few years ago and my doctor didn't bother to tell me if I still had a prostate or, if so, where it had been moved to. Wondering about the particular medical consequences of my surgery and how they're under-researched and under-reported, I note that access to this type of trans-specific health care is a foray into the unknown.

As I return, feeling cut by the assumption that my ever having had a prostate renders me male, I write "#nursingroar" in my notes. This reminds me that I need to return to process this later; that I need to put it out of my body lest it become insidious poison. It's a moment I need to work to unlearn.

Many males do not have prostates and many people with prostates are not male. What my professor espoused is gender essentialism. Our bodies are classified and charted by the medical industrial complex. We are claimed and categorized for the sake of hard science. Rather than defining our own bodies, we are instead defined.

In this instance, using more words to describe phenomena could shift the moment entirely. Rather than saying "every male …" my professor could state "all people with prostates …"[4] This is simple, more accurate, and surreptitiously undoes essentialism. In discussing bodies, not identities, we can allow people to exist in the social world as they choose, while retaining our capacity to understand and address disease processes.

Just as I don't believe that livers are designed, I don't think that my body was somehow a mistake. The "trapped in the wrong body" narrative dominates popular thinking on transness, implying that our bodies are supposed to be a certain way. It implies that our bodies need to be fixed, that we should have the right genitals, the right body fat distribution, the right bone structure, the right vocal pitch, and on and on. This perspective perpetuates a transnormative model of care, by which I mean encouraging us to make our bodies like cis bodies to whatever extent possible, while offering us no other options.

Several years ago, after being on hormones for just over a year, I'd decided I was "cooked." I was exactly what I wanted to be, yet was worried that my body would continue to change. So, after being encouraged by a trans lady friend, I went to my nurse practitioner and told her I didn't want my tiny tits to grow anymore and asked to lower my estrogen dose.

---

4 If you don't know whether your patient has a prostate, try asking over assuming.

She reminded me that there was no research on this, and was miraculously ecstatic about my desires. So we devised a plan, based on her best guess, to play a balancing act with my body. I am my own experiment, because research on what I want for my body has not been done. I can only believe that this is in large part due to direct medical coercion by failing to provide non-binary care and to cissexist standards writ large, because as soon as I started talking about this experience publically, many people that I knew came forward about wanting bodies similarly devalued by the transnormative model of care.

Rather than assuming what trans people want with our bodies, providers could offer options, creating possibilities and access to care. Undoing transnormativity is not solely the burden of trans and genderqueer people. Providers are uniquely situated to help to shift social understandings of gender and bodies and to unburden access to unique and necessary care.

Shifting structures of access and understanding will allow research and care provision to blossom organically. By undermining problematic thinking around trans bodies, we can create a health care system that shifts its focus toward creating agency. This isn't a lost cause or wasted effort. Some are ready to transform their understandings. One professor even started saying "catheterizing a patient with a penis" rather than "a male patient" after recognizing the cissexist implications. Unburdening access to care is as possible as it is necessary.

In my desire to live as an intersex man, I had to decide whether I would try to accommodate the world or make the world accommodate me. I chose the latter because my very life depended on it.

NAVIGATING THIS LIFE AS A BLACK INTERSEX MAN

Sean Saifa Wall

As I sit down to write this narrative, I'm reflecting on the struggle for Black life and sovereignty in the United States. Following the death of Mike Brown in Ferguson, Missouri in the fall of 2014, the United States has seen numerous protests against state-sanctioned and white vigilante violence with the declaration that Black Lives Matter. As a Black intersex man, I have witnessed the impact of state-sanctioned violence on my family and my community, both from the police state and the medical community. I charge them both with state-sanctioned violence, each targeting non-normative bodies—the former through incarceration and execution, the latter by means of surgical and hormonal intervention. As a Black intersex man, I know that this Black body, this intersex body, was not meant to exist. Although this is where I stand now, both socially and politically, I have not always existed here.

I was born in the winter of 1978 at Columbia Presbyterian Hospital in New York City. I was the youngest of five and one of three children in my family who were born with an intersex trait now known as androgen insensitivity syndrome (AIS). At the time, AIS was referred to as "testicular feminization syndrome." AIS is an intersex trait that affects an XY fetus's responsiveness to testosterone in the womb. Upon receiving my medical records at the age of twenty-five, I noticed scribbling and a barrage of notes indicating the process by which the doctors assigned my gender as female. Although I had ambiguous genitalia, which caused some initial confusion among the doctors, XY chromosomes were not enough for me to be raised as male. My mother was told I would be raised as a girl, and the doctor wrote:

> In the interest of proper psychosexual orientation of the infant, and in order to protect the parent's emotional well-being, the mother has been told that:

> The baby is a girl and will function as such.

> She has gonads which require removal in the future (not testes).

Unlike my sisters who were also born with AIS, my mom was not swayed by the surgical recommendations doctors made about my body. As a matter of protocol, my sisters' gonads were removed in infancy; however, my mom made the decision that my testes would remain with me until they had to be removed. My mom told me that the Endocrinology and Pediatric Urology Department at Columbia Presbyterian Hospital hounded her for weeks after I was born, urging her to bring me in for surgery; at every turn, she declined. Although at the time she thought nothing of doing so, her intuition spared me from genital mutilation.

Although I had what doctors refer to as an "enlarged clitoris," I assumed that I was the same as other young women. What I did not learn until I read through my medical records later was that my "enlarged clitoris" was actually a small phallus and my "gonads" were actually undescended testes. Puberty arrived around age eleven and my girl body started to experience a male puberty with broad shoulders, increased body mass, a deep voice, and the beginnings of facial hair. When I was thirteen, my mother took me to see a pediatrician at Columbia Presbyterian because I was experiencing intense pain in my groin area. He suggested that my testes be removed because they could "cause cancer." Within weeks of that visit, I was taken to the children's hospital at Columbia Presbyterian and the surgery was scheduled. The pain that I felt after surgery was perhaps the worst I've experienced in my entire life. After surgery, my pediatrician prescribed estrogen and Provera as a hormonal replacement regimen.

Fatty deposits changed the shape and contours of my face. Once robust and chiseled thighs now harbored cellulite. The beginnings of facial hair and prominent body hair became wispy and nonexistent. What was hard and defined became soft.

At no point did anyone ask me what I wanted to do with my body.

I missed the effects of my natural testosterone such as a deepening voice, increased hair, and muscle mass; when I asked if I could take both testosterone and estrogen after surgery, my mother remarked, "You would look too weird."

The hormone therapy was coupled with intense social conditioning that felt suffocating. When doctors prescribed hormones for me to take, my mother constantly reminded me how "beautiful" the little yellow pills would make me. As a means of reassurance, my pediatrician told my mom that "a lot of fashion models" have AIS and that I would most certainly be beautiful. In our society, gender norms can already be oppressive, but for women with AIS, there is the impact of gender norms and the underlying fear that women with AIS are not really women since they have XY chromosomes. I did not succumb to the pressure to be more feminine, but actually gravitated toward masculinity.

Before transitioning to live as a man, I considered myself a butch woman. When I came out of the closet at fourteen years old and presented as a masculine young woman, I never felt safe. Because I dated women who were more feminine than me, my relationships with them seemed threatening to men who repeatedly reminded me through harassment and threats that I "was not a man." Of course, I wasn't trying to be a man at the time, but it was often an unsavory reminder of how we as a society conflate gender and sexuality.

I grew up as a visibly queer child but I didn't feel different from my peers. What made me feel different were the probing and invasive genital examinations doctors performed on my body. As I got older, the intense scrutiny around my genitals often left me feeling objectified and uncomfortable. Most uncomfortable was that there was never full disclosure of what was happening during these examinations. No one ever explained why they were so interested in my body. I distinctly remember an incident in college where I went to the doctor for a gynecological exam. I had heard stories from my female friends about the speculum and other devices that doctors use to ensure that the reproductive system was functioning normally. Although I was told that I had a "blind vagina" and would never menstruate or have children, I did not fully understand my sexual anatomy. So in the doctor's office, I sat afraid.

When I was brought in, I was asked to disrobe and shortly after, the doctor began her exploration. She stuck a Q-tip inside the orifice and barely managed to get the tip in. She then inserted a finger in my rectum without telling me what she was checking for. This would not be the last time I would be examined anally because doctors were looking for a prostate.

My height, in addition to other features associated with masculinity such as large hands and feet and a deeper voice, blended with a feminine face to create an androgynous presentation. Although I was starting to see myself as more male, I was often frustrated by how estrogen feminized my face and other parts of my body. When I decided to transition from female to male, I was met with resistance from physicians because they incorrectly assumed all people with AIS identify as women. In the beginning of my transition, doctors would often tell me, "I read a chapter on intersex conditions back in medical school," or, "We don't know how to work with people like you" or flat out, "Your body is too weird." Despite these obstacles, I began my transition in early 2004.

I found a home in the transgender male community. Because of the love and support from my trans brothers, I was able to stand firm in my newfound identity as a transgender man. Similar to my friends who were transgender men, once I started testosterone therapy, I experienced heightened sexual arousal, more energy, and a change in how my body stored fat. My partial insensitivity to testosterone meant that I also experienced estrogenic effects such as sore nipples and water retention, which was often frustrating. Because of my inability to produce facial hair and other secondary sex characteristics, I was and sometimes continue to be mistaken for a woman. The doctors who were willing to experiment with dosages were the most supportive of my transition, but they often threw up their hands when my body didn't respond in ways they thought it should.

I wish there was more support for intersex people
to transition to a gender that affirms their identity
if that is their desire.

Although I'm not entirely clear about what testosterone is doing for my body on a cellular level, I will continue to take it because it helps me to feel alive. As my friend Suegee Tamar-Mattis, a doctor specializing in transgender and intersex care, puts it, "You have to put people in the hormonal environment where they feel comfortable."

Today, regardless of how my gender presentation is interpreted, I am either seen as a gay male, a butch woman, or a young man. Despite these variations in how people perceive my gender, more often than not I'm seen in the world as a young Black man. When I transitioned from female to male, I didn't feel the same level of vulnerability I felt as a masculine-of-center queer woman who dated feminine women. Prior to transition, I felt scared and was often harassed and disrespected, and at times feared for my physical safety. Now my fear is something that stretches back to the annals of American history from the time when Black men were once lynched with abandon until today when we are imprisoned in disproportionate numbers. As a Black intersex man, I am fearful of getting arrested and being subject to strip searches where once again my genitals would be on display in an institutional setting that is inherently violent. I am now navigating this world as a Black intersex man.

In my desire to live as an intersex man, I had to decide whether I would try to accommodate the world or make the world accommodate me. I chose the latter because my very life depended on it.

I am realizing that my Black intersex body is a site of resistance. I am putting my body and life experiences on the line as an intersex activist because I want to create a world in which people born with variations of sexual anatomy are free to live with dignity and respect. I am advocating for a world where intersex children can enjoy body autonomy and where the uniqueness of their bodies, and our bodies as intersex adults, are upheld in their integrity and beauty. I am advocating for a world where we are meant to exist.

I continually question my own motives and rationalizations. I've told myself that it is a reality that there are gates, and someone has to be there to open them. But why not work to destroy these gates? Am I no different from the people who acted as gatekeepers in early gender clinics?

CONFESSIONS OF A GENDER SPECIALIST

Sand C. Chang

I have GID. Not Gender Identity Disorder (though this is arguable), but Gatekeeper Identity Disorder. Which side of the gate am I on? Both. Pause. Let's get the introductions out of the way. I am: Chinese American, genderqueer, gender fluid, queer, generation X, Capricorn, nonreligious spiritual, upper middle class, a psychologist, a dancer, a foodie, and a small dog enthusiast. (Note: Order and contents subject to change depending on social context.) On second thought, there is no way to get these aspects of my experience out of the way. They pave the roads that lead to either side of the gate. I never thought to myself, "When I grow up I want to be a Gender Specialist," but here I am. So how did I get here, you ask?

My formal education as a psychologist never offered opportunities for coursework related to gender identity. I focused my studies on psychoanalysis, addictions, eating disorders, and racial identity. Discussions concerning gender focused exclusively on the binary options of man/male/masculine and woman/female/feminine. This was the early 2000s, and while there is now slightly more awareness, things haven't changed much in psychology graduate training. My passion and commitment to advocacy for transgender and gender nonconforming (TGNC) people within mental health practice has more or

45

less been viewed as some strange side interest that does not truly concern most clinicians.

Things were different in my personal life where I became steeped in learning about TGNC people, identities, and experiences. People in my community, including friends and partners, were starting to transition, and when I came across the concept of genderqueer and nonbinary identities, something resonated in me. I am grateful to the many TGNC activists, artists, writers, scholars, and friends, many of whom were people of colour, who took part in my politicization process and schooled me in challenging the dominant narratives around TGNC health and identity. I learned that this house was never built for us, but we have been expected to abide by its rules.

My therapist at the time (with whom I had a codependent relationship) was not pleased. She became very uncomfortable when I started to question gender. And when I shared for the first time that I was dating a trans man, she outright said, "You don't want to get involved with *those people*. They have a lot of trauma." Little did I know that this one statement would somehow characterize many upcoming challenges in my career as an advocate for TGNC health within the field of psychology.

I moved to New York in 2005 to intern at a college counseling center and started facilitating trainings on gender identity. Here I began to feel the pressure of tokenization as a gender nonconforming person of colour. Shortly after, I was lucky enough to secure an externship at the Gender Identity Project (GIP) at the New York LGBT Center, where all staff members had a TGNC identity. What was most beautiful about this experience was not that I felt affirmed in my genderqueer identity, but that I felt ordinary. It felt good to blend in, to have my gender be nothing special, to not have the lonely experience of being a token. It was powerful to see TGNC people in leadership positions, and it set me up to demand that TGNC voices be heard in health care.

Returning to California in 2008, it was difficult to be back in predominantly white cisgender work environments. I chose not to be out as genderqueer in those settings, preferring that others just not know, rather than them being unwilling to respectfully deal with my genderqueer identity. Experiences of racism, sexism, transphobia, and ageism (due to looking ten years younger than my age) led me to believe that I couldn't be taken seriously unless I wore binary drag and passed as cisgender to my colleagues. Was this a fear of discrimination or survival instinct? Probably both.

When I started my private practice, I didn't set out to specialize in working with other TGNC folks (in fact, part of me resisted it in order to preserve my personal life), but TGNC clients found me because I was one of few therapists in the area who listed "transgender" as a population I work with. It still wasn't too popular to be interested in TGNC health, not like it's become now. Doing psychotherapy, helping people to feel empowered in their authentic identities, was what was rewarding about the job. Writing letters for doctors and surgeons was my least favorite part, and I had to grapple with what it meant to be a gatekeeper, whether I liked it or not.

Despite my political objections to the diagnosis, I found myself documenting Gender Identity Disorder so that my clients could access services. I refused to join the World Professional Association for Transgender Health (WPATH) because I didn't agree with the classism, racism, sexism, homophobia, and cisgender bias and privilege embedded in their excessive requirements for people seeking medical transition. The ideal candidate for hormones or surgery was typically one that resembled those with evaluative power (i.e., white, cisnormative, heteronormative) and had the ability to pay out-of-pocket. I refused to be part of an organization that didn't centre the voices of TGNC people in their own health care. Still, I found myself complying with WPATH standards by writing the letters my clients were asking for. Years later, I've started to engage in conversations with WPATH members because I have seen progress, especially with the most recent Standards of Care released in 2011. But I'm an impatient motherfucker, and sometimes, most of the time, it's just not enough.

Throughout my career, I have grappled with how to align the gatekeeping role with my values and ethics. From the start, I make it clear that I have a dual role: first and foremost, as a therapist who can provide emotional support and psychoeducation with a consideration of the client's long-term best interest, and second, as an evaluator of the request for hormones or surgery. I tell prospective clients that I will provide a letter no matter what, but that what I can include in the letter is dependent on a detailed conversation about information and expectations concerning the requested medical intervention. I talk about the power imbalance and acknowledge my role as a gatekeeper. I am transparent about my disagreement with the necessity of diagnoses, yet willingly document Gender Dysphoria when necessary (i.e., when it will help the client achieve their goals). And I tell them that, letter aside, I am interested in supporting them in their process should they need it. I believe that everyone needs to have a support system in place while undergoing transition, and a therapist may or may not be part of that system. This approach is by no means perfect, and I hope that I always have enough humility to consider it a work in progress.

I continually question my own motives and rationalizations. I've told myself that it is a reality that there are gates, and someone has to be there to open them. But why not work to destroy these gates? Am I no different from the people who acted as gatekeepers in early gender clinics? As health professionals, many of them thought they were doing good. I may not be scrutinizing people for a convincing gender story (e.g., I couldn't care less what kind of childhood toys a person played with), but I'm still evaluating the capacity to provide informed consent. Is this a way of disguising the gates? Or just making them invisible? I may tell myself that I can change the system from within, but maybe the system is so broken that it needs to be abandoned. Maybe we need to start over, and participating in the system now is only keeping it alive. Are these small, incremental wins in access to TGNC health care truly progress, or are they distractions that simply placate and thus prevent revolutionary change and true liberation?

There's also the issue of what I'm calling "dual otherness"—being both the gatekeeper and part of the community. How this plays out in my life and work is that among other gatekeepers (i.e., doctors, surgeons, therapists), I'm not always taken seriously because I'm perceived as having in-group bias or advocating too hard for affirming care. And with clients and sometimes other members of TGNC communities, I may be viewed as the enemy. Other TGNC folks don't always see me as similar to them, either because my genderqueer identity/expression doesn't qualify me for *real* TGNC status (whatever that means), because I have class and education privilege that affords me a position of power, because my versions of masculinity and femininity fuck with the very white and medicalized ideals and narratives that these concepts are based on, and because I will never know what it's like to be in their shoes. That's fair; my privilege in this dynamic is undeniable. I am suspicious of my own narcissistic need to be seen as "good" in these contexts.

Something I struggle with the most is how the power that mental health professionals have historically had over TGNC people's lives has created a huge barrier for TGNC people who want support from a therapist. When TGNC people have to fight so hard to resist being labeled as sick, it can get in the way of being able to ask for help when it is truly needed. The result is further stigma of mental illness. It's a form of ableism. When TGNC people say, "I'm not mentally ill," it can be empowering. It can also be othering and shaming of anyone who does have mental illness. It can make it impossible for anyone who has experienced trauma to find the healing they need. The key factor here is choice. I want anyone who wants services to feel the freedom to access them, and I don't want it to be forced upon anyone.

Working in TGNC health care, I've always got my guard up. The microaggressions (or macroaggressions) can be around every corner of an otherwise casual conversation. And it hurts. It's personal. I have to do a lot of self-care. I try to name what's happening around me, make what's behind these gates more transparent. So here it is, my ever-growing list of problematic dynamics witnessed on a regular basis in TGNC health care:

1   Minimizing challenges that TGNC people face by comparing us to cisgender people. Example: "I know it's hard that we can't change your name in our computer system, but women who get married and change their last name have to deal with this too."

2   This phone call: "Do you have ten minutes to teach me how to work with TGNC people?" This diminishes the lived experiences of TGNC people and devalues me as a genderqueer health professional.

3   Locking the gates (e.g., saying "no" to a request for surgery) because someone doesn't have housing or adequate support. I feel strongly in these cases that the answer shouldn't be "no" but "let's talk about what we need to do to get you prepared."

4   Locking the gates because someone doesn't fit the medicalized narrative (e.g., didn't become aware of their TGNC identity until adulthood).

5   Locking the gates because someone has trauma or assuming that trauma caused a TGNC identity. In a society that constantly delegitimizes and inflicts violence upon TGNC folks and their bodies, who the hell doesn't have trauma? Being traumatized shouldn't be a barrier; it should be a sign that someone needs help.

6   Heterosexism, misogyny, and scrutiny about how people use their genitals. Comments like, "His sexual practices are very … different" make me ask, "Different from what?"

7   Denying medical necessity, assuming requested procedures are cosmetic, yet requiring a mental health diagnosis. The term "cosmetic" has no place in these conversations, as it inevitably leads to comparisons with cisgender people having the same procedures.

8   When I've advocated for TGNC people to be in leadership in TGNC health care settings, I've gotten passive responses equaling something to the effect of, "That would be nice, I guess." There is no true commitment to making this happen. I once brought it up on a professional listserv and was told that this notion was discriminatory against cisgender people.

9   Ageism/adultism plays out not only toward TGNC youth, but toward TGNC adults who often look younger than they are. This is used as an excuse to question the validity of a TGNC person's identity or decision-making capacity.

10 TGNC people as a "career opportunity." Providers have said this to me about their own fortuitous landings in positions of power in TGNC health care, while others have said it to me as if I've struck gold. That's not why I do the work. TGNC people don't want to be considered career advancement or money-making opportunities. We want to be seen as people who deserve affirming and competent medical care like anyone else.

11 Gatekeeping for gatekeepers. There is a push for certification of gender specialists. While I'm all for competent care and increased education, I don't think any certification can guarantee a culturally competent and affirming experience. I admit to being guilty of this one myself. Because I have seen a lot of harm done to TGNC folks by incompetent providers, I have a list of trusted colleagues who I refer TGNC people to for services. When it's already difficult for TGNC people, poor people, and people of colour to access education and licensure, requiring certification would further systematically bar these people from providing care to their communities. It's those communities that would suffer.

12 When TGNC folks complain about the shitty care they're receiving and demand change, providers point to their mental health diagnoses as a way to discount their concerns. This is a way of putting TGNC people in their places and making it known who has the power. It communicates that compliance is the only way to get one's needs met. My view is that self-advocacy is a sign of good mental health and the resilience to fight against oppressive systems. We know we deserve better.

13 Equating "TGNC health care" with medical transition. This denies the other medical needs of TGNC folks. My vision of quality TGNC health care is the idea that a TGNC person (of any background) could walk into any medical office (e.g., dermatology, oncology) and receive respectful and competent care.

All of this tells me that my work is cut out for me. So I struggle and I ask these questions. I get angry and scared when I don't see others around me asking themselves the same questions. And then I reach for my community and tap into my own resources so that I can keep fighting, with myself, with other providers, with systems that cause harm. For me, the remedy for this Gatekeeper Identity Disorder is to be painfully aware of it, to never let myself think that I'm cured.

My visits to the clinic also put in relief how easy it is to get lost in the health care system. One physician, nurse, or social worker knows a fragment of you, a version, and knows a fraction of what you did with the other health caregivers, all coordinated computer systems notwithstanding. There has never been a time in which we are so connected by technology—the fast and furious digitization of your Self—and so shipwrecked and lost in it.

READ THIS BEFORE YOUR NEXT CLINICAL VISIT

Cheap Advice for Frequent Patients

Francisco Ibàñez-Carrasco

Two strangers and I sit in front of a high resolution screen. In it, a round solar asteroid is ablaze. It is a bright disk of crimson, furious molten gold, and tangerine. There are craters and viscous eruptions of lava. I have put my clothes back on and some of my dignity. I have wiped myself as best as I could. I hold my head up high and I am here engaging in nearly casual conversation about the pixellated asteroid presence of my anus on a monitor.

The medical gaze separates my quirky self from my patient self. My anus has its own cinemascope production on display. Watching the screen, we are all spectators at a safe distance from my excretory system. An audience sheltered from this devoted and irrational male flytrap of seed. The conversation is always about the technical malfunction of the former, about what is wrong with me.

These anal dysplasia clinic visits have been, for over ten years, one of my most enigmatic and disassociating medical appointments. More detaching than pulling my Self apart with mental health caregivers to exteriorize my shame and fear of sex, to connect those childhood disembodiments with my love of dick and, apparently, my extreme sexual interests. And even to study the disconnections between my health and my professional life as an HIV researcher.

People who get pap smears or STI tests probably understand what it is to have a no-strings-attached, nearly casual, and sometimes alarming conversation about a sex organ with a stranger. A stranger who has the power of an oracle to deliver bad news. And at least in my case, a stranger who douses your anal canal with vinegar to make visible your precancerous or cancerous cells or lesions. (You squirming yet?) A stranger who on occasion biopsies your insides, which is like having a fat ant biting you treacherously. A stranger who can burn inside you with a laser gun. Zap!

To distract myself from this aloof mortification of the flesh, I think of fabulousness—a comforting gay illusion. I think of Farrah Fawcett; she had anal cancer. But I digress ...

The anal dysplasia clinic puts me on display for the medical system— and I have been on display at many clinics. I was photographed naked every week for a research study at the Cancer Agency in Vancouver in 1994 when I had advanced Kaposi's sarcoma, for example. The anal dysplasia clinic highlights the modernity of clinical care, with their efficiency designed to reduce shame and surprise.

Upon reflection on my well-established experience (indeed, unrecognized expertise) as patient in this and other clinics I have to visit frequently all over the city, I see the superb role that technology plays and how it continues to de-skill physicians, albeit not disempowering them. Much like the neat screen at the anal dysplasia clinic, technology and media now permeate most health interactions. We do not know what it will do to our interactions in the long term—maybe the same it has done for gay sex?

My visits to the clinic also put in relief how easy it is to get lost in the health care system. One physician, nurse, or social worker knows a fragment of you, a version, and knows a fraction of what you did with the other health caregivers, all coordinated computer systems notwithstanding. There has never been a time in which we are so connected by technology—the fast and furious digitization of your Self—and so shipwrecked and lost in it.

No wonder patients need "peer navigators" these days to help us plot a course in the labyrinthine health services. My experience as an HIV-positive person since 1986 is that the health care system has gradually become more fragmented. "The system," this byzantine accumulation of forms, bureaucratic procedures, auscultations, prodding of cold metallic objects in all orifices, prescriptions, adverse side-effects, confusing buildings and soul-crushing coloured offices with the fatidic signalling of brutal cryptograms, intakes and exits, seems effective and friendly from my privileged white Latino, overeducated standpoint. It would be hypocritical to cry foul. However, it would be indolent to deny that the system is unfair and obscenely offensive to many, especially those who chronically or episodically present complex needs: transgender folks, those at odds with the law, illicit drug users, or people with episodic conditions such as MS or mood disorders. I get that.

I saw one general practitioner for twenty-two years since my HIV diagnosis; he is seventy-seven and retired about ten years ago. He saw too much of AIDS and burned out. He recently wrote me a letter in which he tells me the only "gay" he sees and does these days is his partner and some porn. He read my memoir, *Giving It Raw*, and realized I am his friend, an ex-patient, one of the few left.

And this is my biggest piece of advice from over thirty years in the health care system in Canada and brief visitations to other health care systems (when I have been travelling and I've been ill) and my work as researcher in the field: make friends fast. This might not be "the remedy," but your ability to communicate your story, to relate to the stranger(s) in front of you is probably the one most immediate tool you have. And you have a small window of opportunity. Use it wisely to establish a relationship.

Unfortunately, working with health care providers is redolent of going to job interviews. It is anxiety-producing to be interviewed by one or a group that has technical knowledge and the petty bureaucratic power to deploy it. The first impression you make and your clear answers to exactly what you're being asked are crucial.

In this context of disparity, you are encouraged and sometimes required to have a voice, to be an assertive consumer of health care services. They will tell you that, in this neoliberal market of health brands and services, you can make choices—the way you choose your tooth paste—and this is simply not the case. The choices are limited by the tiered health system in Canada (never "universal"), what privilege you have or how proficient you are as a patient (never impatient). For starters, there is a language of wellness and survivorship and victimhood—all in one incongruous melange—a health literacy that you are expected to master.

Living with HIV through its dark 1980s and 1990s decades and the new normalized age of HIV as a chronic manageable (albeit stigmatized and criminalized) medical condition has forced me to adopt and adapt this discourse. Being a radical and using an antagonistic discourse would send me into a rapid collision course with many administrators, medics, and specialists. I had to find "my voice" inside the cavernous voice of the master. I have to ventriloquate the established edicts and maxims in order to slip in my queer needs. At the anal dysplasia clinic, we talk about human papillomavirus (HPV) and high grade pre-cancerous cells. We never talk about fisting properly or enhancing the experience of anal pleasure.

And there is the petty but aggravating plebeian revenge of the masses, also known as the internet. This is the medusa feared by health care providers. We know all the language they know and more. If you can find the recipe for a terrorist bomb online, you can find the recipe for your cure, right? Patients are gathered in guerrilla cells such as Patients Like Me, the patient-powered research network. They come to their appointments with questions and requests and diagrams that only schooled patients would have had thirty years ago. It is a minor sinister pleasure to see the widened eyes and twirling pupils of a doc when you have done your homework and bring it out of the box.

We "patients" have something archetypal in us—we are the rabid activist who never lets down their guard and protests everything (the squeaky wheel gets the grease), the fastidious internet-learned who knows every single clinical and scientific fact about their illness, and the victim who thinks they deserve nothing at all and lets the health system trample all over them. Each one of the many who populate a waiting room has something we can learn from. Navigating the health system is a form of askesis, an everyday training to be an athlete. Medical patients train like athletes. We exercise self-discipline or self-control, if not always for religious or meditative purposes, to obtain what (we think) we need.

My advice to you, gleaned from my experiences as a frequent patient? Learn about the medical system, your illness, your health care providers, your rights and responsibilities (but do not obsess like I sometimes do). Some resistance is futile, some is warranted. Make the homework you have done visible to your health care providers without cracking their at times fragile egos. Understand them as technicians with great gadgets and pharmaceuticals, be afraid of their petty administrative power (because they use it), treat each new interaction as a job interview, make good friends, find your voice within the voice of the master.

Remember: story often trumps data and our health is not the accumulation of arbitrary numbers from tests. Live to tell in your voice the things from your personal experiences that intersect with the clinical language, the clinical facts, this other Frankenstein persona they compose about you in charts and graphs. Your quest for survival is to stay human and compassionate in the throes of rampant medicalization.

QUEER AND TRANS HEALTH INNOVATION PROFILE

The Q Card Project (Seattle, Washington)

Genya Shimkin, MPH, Founder

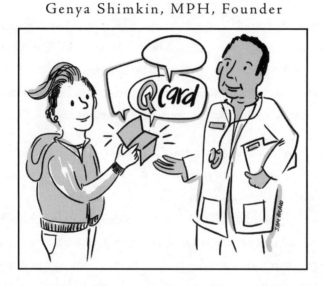

Tell us about the Q Card Project and why you're proud of it.

In its most basic form, the Q Card is a simple and easy-to-use communication tool designed to empower queer and trans youth and educate and support their health care providers. Designed with input from queer youth, health care providers, youth advocates, and community organizers, the Q Card is a tri-fold business card that allows youth to fill in their sexual orientation, gender identity, preferred gender pronouns, and any specific concerns. It also offers tips on how to provide more sensitive care to queer and trans youth, and lists a number of documented health disparities in the LGBTQ community.

What changes are you trying to create? What problems are you trying to solve? What does success look like?

I want to live in a world where all queer, trans, and gender nonconforming people have access to quality, sensitive health care that validates their experiences, and where they can achieve wellness whatever that looks like for them.

I don't know a single queer or trans person who hasn't had a crummy experience in health care—those range from microinvalidations and microaggressions all the way to assault by health care providers. We can't continue to be okay with this as the status quo. I want to empower people to have a voice and to create change from within the system.

If someone from another place emailed you to say, "I want to do this in my community," and asked for your advice on how to do it, what would you tell them?

Talk to your community. The Q Card wouldn't have worked if I wrote it myself. I have all this privilege: I'm a white woman with a graduate degree, and I'm older than the youth the card is intended for. When I first drafted the card, I brought it to queer and trans youth to ask them what they would change about it, and their input made the card and the format relatable to the people it was intended for. For example, the first prototype was an 8.5 x 11" sheet of paper folded in half. The youth I showed it to said it needed to be small enough to fit into their wallets. If I hadn't talked to them early on I might've created something that wasn't usable.

Right now we're working on getting the card translated into Spanish. Instead of hiring a professional translator, I hired a group of queer and trans youth who speak Spanish as a first language to translate the card into language that resonates with them.

At every step of the way I go back to the youth who've become ambassadors for the Q Card. We've built connections and community from the ground up. I'm endlessly impressed by the way that the youth I work with are able to help me reframe things and think in new ways.

If the Q Card Project was gifted $1 million (with no strings attached) by a donor, and your success was completely guaranteed, what would you choose to do?

I would use it as seed money to build an LGBTQ centre of health excellence in Seattle. The clinic would be part of a community centre that also had a dedicated LGBTQ youth homeless shelter. It would offer services for everyone regardless of income, including sliding scale services and access to medications.

Is there anything else you'd like to tell us?

The project has totally exploded in ways I never could've imagined, in large part because of the people who've stepped up to offer their support and expertise, to check me on stuff, and to teach me.

My favourite thing is when someone I've just met asks me, "Hey, have you heard about the Q Card?" People feel genuine ownership of it, and it's being used in ways I never could have imagined—like the therapist who gives them to queer and trans youth for their teachers to help the youth feel safer in the classroom.

This project started as a goofy idea I had as a grad student, and it's become the beating heart of my life's work. This is not where I thought my life was going to be and I'm so happy. I'm incredibly lucky.

**For more information about the Q Card Project,
visit qcardproject.com**

Whether implicit or explicit, bias and discrimination perpetuate shame and stigma in the clinical environment and can be (re)traumatizing—particularly for populations that experience higher levels of stress, adversity, and health disparities. In order to encourage individuals to take charge of their health and autonomize their own health care decisions, these negative interpersonal interactions must be addressed, including training physicians to be competent in caring for lesbian, gay, bisexual, and transgender patients.

USING MEDICAL EDUCATION TO ADVANCE HEALTH OF LGBT INDIVIDUALS

Kristen L. Eckstrand

Do they know what *they're talking about? Will they act nicely? What will they think of me? Will they be professional?* These are common questions that many patients ask themselves when going to the doctor. The questions seem simple enough, but knowing, thinking, acting, and being reflect complex paradigms of knowledge, attitudes, skills, and behaviours addressed by medical education. What becomes the "felt" experience of patients when receiving care from a doctor reflects what medical educators refer to as "competence"—an observable ability of a health professional, integrating multiple components such as knowledge, skills, values, and attitudes. Examples of this are demonstrating accountability to LGBT patients, society, and the profession by accepting shared responsibility for eliminating disparities and overt bias, and developing policies and procedures that respect all patients' rights to self-determination.

63

Yet negative interpersonal experiences in health care, particularly as they relate to sexual orientation, gender identity, and gender expression, persist.[1] These sometimes manifest as explicit bias, such as refusing to let someone's same-sex partner into a care area or using inappropriate language, but they're more often experienced as implicit bias or microaggressions. Such unconscious patterns of behaviour or communication are not consciously intended to be discriminatory, but nonetheless cause harm, like misgendering someone or not taking a sexual history when relevant to the clinical encounter. Whether implicit or explicit, bias and discrimination perpetuate shame and stigma in the clinical environment and can be (re)traumatizing—particularly for populations that experience higher levels of stress, adversity, and health disparities.[2] In order to encourage individuals to take charge of their health and autonomize their own health care decisions, these negative interpersonal interactions must be addressed, including training physicians to be competent in caring for LGBT patients.

Previous projects developed by experts in LGBT health tackled developing curricular recommendations[3], but their uptake in medical

1 J.M. Grant, et al., *Injustice at Every Turn: A Report of the National Transgender Discrimination Survey* (Washington, DC: National Center for Transgender Equality, 2011); Institute of Medicine, *The Health of Lesbian, Gay, Bisexual, and Transgender People: Building a Foundation for Better Understanding* (Washington: Institute of Medicine, 2011); Lambda Legal, *When Health Care Isn't Caring: Lambda Legal's Survey of Discrimination Against LGBT People and People with HIV* (New York: Lambda Legal, 2010); H.J. Makadon et al., *Fenway Guide to Lesbian, Gay, Bisexual, and Transgender Health*, 2nd ed. (Philadelphia: American College of Physicians, 2015).

2 Institute of Medicine, 2011.

3 American Academy of Child and Adolescent Psychiatry, "Practice parameter on gay, lesbian, or bisexual sexual orientation, gender nonconformity, and gender discordance in children and adolescents," *Journal of the American Academy of Child & Adolescent Psychiatry* 51, no. 9 (2012): 957-74; J. Satterfield and the UCSF Chancellor's GLBT Issues Advisory Sub-Committee on Curriculum, *UCSF Tool for Assessing Cultural Competence Training–LGBT Adaptations*, unpublished report.

education has been minimal. Their recommended additions to physician training addressed critically relevant topics in LGBT health, but the recommendations were hard to integrate into required curricula because they didn't fit the structure of existing medical training—Competency-Based Medical Education (CBME). CBME is an outcomes-based approach to the design, implementation, assessment of learners, and the evaluation of medical education programs, using an organizing framework of competencies. But they were viewed as extraneous or too time-intensive for an already dense curriculum.[4]

As a member of the LGBT community, a medical educator, and a young physician, I initially felt disheartened to learn that education that could improve and even save lives is omitted from curricula for such trivial reasons. My perspective changed when I came to see working with the CBME framework as a strategy to advance LGBT content in medical curricula. Grounding the competencies required to care for patients of diverse sexual orientations and gender identities in a broadly utilized framework represented one solution to the lack of integration of LGBT content in medical education.

CBME, the format for current, international medical education curricula and the necessary framework in which to develop proficiency in addressing LGBT health, is relatively new compared to the history of the medical profession. Understanding why medical education operates using this education structure is critical for understanding the importance of implementing change for medical curricula.

Medical education's history is rich and independent, but is also influenced by concurrent changes in societal and scientific thought. Prior

---

4 Juno Obedin-Maliver, et al., "Lesbian, gay, bisexual, and transgender–related content in undergraduate medical education." JAMA 306, no. 9 (2011): 971-77; Rebecca L. Tamas, et al., "Addressing patient sexual orientation in the undergraduate medical education curriculum," *Academic Psychiatry* 34, no. 5 (2010): 342-45.

to 1910, medical education was unstandardized, variable, often for-profit, and implemented with minimal oversight. Abraham Flexner's 1910 report, *Medical Education in the United States and Canada*, called for a new system of academic medicine emphasizing education and scientific discovery alongside patient care. The educational framework imposed became known as "Structure/Process" education, where all medical schools taught a fixed four-year curriculum with a dedicated amount of time and format given to each discipline (anatomy, psychiatry, surgery, etc.).

Several challenges arose to Flexnerian thinking over the past century: research advances in biomedical and clinical sciences exponentially increased the amount of "knowledge" embedded in curricula; high-profile cases of physician abuses of power and unethical practices demonstrated the importance of including ethics in training; an increase in attention to the need to account for diversity, including sexual orientation and gender identity, in clinical practice; and a shift towards insurance-based models of payment for health care in efforts to try and balance excessive spending with ensuring access to care for all. Growing dissatisfaction with health care and medical providers led to a demand for responsibility and accountability—medical education had to respond.[5]

The result was a paradigm shift from Structure/Process education to Competency-Based Medical Education.[6] Rather than the "fixed time, variable outcome" Structure/Process educational model, CBME emphasized a "variable time, fixed outcome" format where the ultimate outcome is physician competence. Understanding CBME requires a basic familiarity with its core terminology.

---

5 Carol Carraccio, et al., "Shifting paradigms: from Flexner to competencies," *Academic Medicine* 77, no. 5 (2002): 361-67; Jason R. Frank et al., "Competency-based medical education: theory to practice," Medical Teacher 32, no. 8 (2010): 638-45.

6 Jason R. Frank and Deborah Danoff, "The CanMEDS initiative: implementing an outcomes-based framework of physician competencies," *Medical Teacher* 29, no. 7 (2007): 642-47.

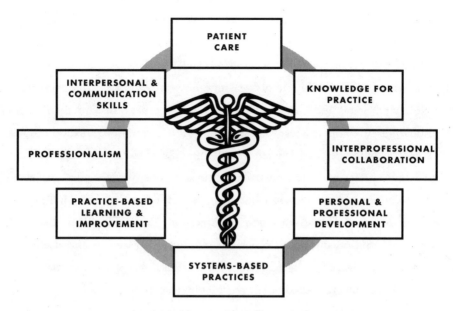

Figure 1. Domains of Competence of the Physician Competency Reference Set, in which outcome competencies are delineated.

Some I've already discussed, such as "competence" and the definition of CBME. Entrustable professional activity (EPA) is the essential day-to-day activities of a specialty or a profession that an individual must be trusted to perform without direct supervision (e.g., performing a complete and sensitive history and physical exam on a transgender patient). Domain of Competence is the broad distinguishable areas of proficiency that, in the aggregate, constitute a general descriptive structure for a profession (see Figure 1). Finally, a milestone is a defined, observable marker of an individual's ability along a developmental continuum (e.g., applying guidelines for gender-affirming hormone therapy).

CBME is implemented via four components: identifying the outcomes, defining performance levels (milestones) for each competency, assessing proficiency in a developmental structure, and continuous evaluation to ensure the desired outcomes are met.[7] As CBME gained traction in medical education, so too did the number of expected curricular outcomes that educators developed. When the Association of American Medical Colleges (an organization representing the medical schools, teaching hospitals, and academic societies of the United States and Canada) embarked on the process of simplifying them, thousands of "competencies" were being taught across various medical schools. This array, while well intentioned, created unnecessary redundancy and difficulty in defining performance levels, particularly in areas where fewer clinical guidelines and recommendations are available, such as LGBT health. Through a process of careful review, the Association of American Medical Colleges identified, simplified, and organized outcomes into the Physician Competency Reference Set—a standardized set of fifty-eight competencies across eight domains (see Figure 1) defining the outcomes in general physician training.[8]

There are also a vast number of milestones. These are used in undergraduate medical training (medical school) and graduate medical training (residency and fellowship) to understand what level a trainee is performing at and whether additional training in certain areas is necessary to support competence.[9] Milestones, unlike the competencies in the Reference Set, have yet to be fully standardized across the training continuum. International initiatives have been helpful in defining performance levels for graduate medical education in different medical specialties (surgery, psychiatry, etc.) but no universal milestones are available for undergraduate medical education relating to the Reference Set.

7 Carraccio, et al., 2002.

8 Robert Englander, et al., "Toward a common taxonomy of competency domains for the health professions and competencies for physicians," *Academic Medicine* 88, no. 8 (2013): 1088-94.

9 Susan R. Swing, "The ACGME outcome project: retrospective and prospective," *Medical Teacher* 29, no. 7 (2007): 648-54.

Entrustable professional activities are emerging as the assessment framework for undergraduate medical education and are currently being tested at medical schools in the United States.[10] These consist of a simple "Yes/No" decision where a medical student does/does not perform a core entrustable professional activity (e.g., taking a complete history and performing a physical exam) required to participate in clinical practice without direct supervision (e.g., as a resident physician). Each one requires proficiency in multiple domains. A failure of this can be linked back to competence in a developmental framework because each activity is defined by certain Reference Set competencies. That means targeted educational interventions can be provided to learners in order to become entrustable with all patients, including those with diverse sexual orientations and gender identities.

This overriding framework on competence has helped standardize education towards achieving the expected outcomes of physician training—including culturally responsive care inclusive of sexual orientation, gender identity, and gender expression.

The Physician Competency Reference Set is a standardized taxonomy defining the outcomes required of a twenty-first-century physician. These are abstract and not contextual (e.g., interacting with a person who is LGBT). For example, one Reference Set competency in the Patient Care domain of competence states that physicians should be able to "Gather essential and accurate information about patients and their conditions through history-taking, physical examination, and the use of laboratory data, imaging, and other tests." Here, "patient" describes any individual receiving medical care irrespective of their background, identity, or ability. The data discussed earlier about LGBT individuals' experiences in health

10 O. ten Cate, "Entrustability of professional activities and competency-based training," *Medical Education* 39, no. 12 (2005): 1176-7. doi: 10.1111/j.1365-2929.2005.02341.x.ten Cate; AAMC, 2014a

care indicates that some physicians aren't proficient in this area, suggesting a need for clarifying the Reference Set when context-specific needs of populations are not being met.

To remedy this, the Association of American Medical Colleges convened an Advisory Committee on Sexual Orientation, Gender Identity, and Sex Development in 2012. The charge of the committee was to create competencies to support the training of medical students to care for patients of diverse sexual orientations and gender identities. Understanding that previous attempts lacked widespread uptake, the committee decided to ground their training recommendations in the existing CBME framework—the Physician Competency Reference Set.

Providing context to the Reference Set to improve training in caring for LGBT patients began by determining which Reference Set competencies required qualification and which competencies a student could be expected to perform when caring for an LGBT patient without any additional training. For example, one competency that does not require qualification comes from the Personal and Professional Development domain—"Manage conflict between personal and professional responsibilities." It should be possible to demonstrate this in any context.

However, the Patient Care competency—"Gather essential and accurate information about patients and their conditions through history taking, physical examination, and the use of laboratory data, imaging, and other tests"—does require additional context. Health and wellness for individuals who are LGBT depend on the providers' ability to clinically elicit and address the topics, including sexual orientation, gender identity, and sex development—and proficiency is lacking in this area.[11] To include this context, the committee qualified the aforementioned

11 Nelson F. Sanchez, et al., "Medical Students' Ability to Care for Lesbian, Gay, Bisexual, and Transgendered Patients," *Family Medicine* 38, no. 1 (2006): 21-7;.Yolanda H. Wimberly et al., "Sexual history-taking among primary care physicians," *Journal of the National Medical Association* 98, no. 12 (2006): 1924.

competency by adding the statement, "... by sensitively and effectively eliciting relevant information about sex anatomy, sex development, sexual behavior, sexual history, sexual orientation, sexual identity, and gender identity from all patients in a developmentally appropriate manner." Not only does this qualifier identify key terminology and core concepts for use in teaching, the language also supports the assessment of trainee competence.

This process of identifying gaps in performance, determining which competencies require additional context, and developing qualifiers to address gaps is iterative; of the fifty-eight competencies of the Physician Competency Reference Set, twenty were determined to need additional qualification, and thirty qualifiers were developed to address known gaps. The Association of American Medical Colleges published these qualifiers, the first adaptation of the Reference Set, in 2014.[12]

Adapting the Physician Competency Reference Set is the first step to inclusive and effective medical education designed to meet the needs of patients who identify as LGBT by defining the outcome competencies (and qualifiers). Subsequent work must build on these qualifiers within the Competency-Based Medical Education framework to define performance levels for each qualifier, assess qualifiers in a developmental framework, and implement continuous evaluation to ensure the desired outcomes are met. These efforts must extend beyond undergraduate medical education into training and evaluating current providers—including nurse practitioners, physician assistants, pharmacists, and other members of health care teams—so as to effect the necessary change across the entire health care system in order to ensure the health and well-being of patients with diverse sexual orientations, gender identities, and sex developments.

---

12 Association of American Medical Colleges, *Implementing curricular and climate changes to improve health care for individuals who are LGBT, gender nonconforming, or born with DSD* (Washington, DC, 2014b).

Let me stress this point: I did my own research. The doctors did not help. The
information I found was from personal sources telling their own stories and shar-
ing what they found. I don't love the idea of crowdsourcing my own health and
wellness, getting solutions to medical problems on Tumblr, but with a body that's
an unknown in the medical system, what else was I supposed to do?

HEALTH AS A SPIRITUAL PRACTICE

Or, Please Don't Call Me "Lady"

Sinclair Sexsmith

"Miss! You need to fill out one more form," as someone waves a clipboard.

"Right this way, young lady," as I'm shown to the exam room.

"Have you been here before, ma'am?" as I check in.

I can't go for more than five minutes of an interaction with the medical industry without being gendered female. Immediately, I am defensive. Immediately, I am dysphoric. Immediately, after each time they use terms like "lady" and "miss" and "ma'am," the message is clear: They do not understand my body. So why would I trust them to help me with my health and wellness?

I've generally been "healthy," or at least that's what I always heard from doctors during annual exams. All my tests looked good. My body checked out. I've never had conversations about genderqueerness with my health practitioners—until the past two years. About that time, everything about my health changed, and it took me seeking care from four different practitioners in four modalities to get a real diagnosis and start feeling healthier again.

I moved from New York City to the San Francisco Bay Area in 2013.

About six months later, I felt so different—the stress of living in such a chaotic, high-energy, high-consequence city started falling away. That's when I began noticing big fluctuations in my moods that were connected to my menstrual cycle, and started to seek support and help to see what was happening. I've had heavy periods for years, since my twenties, with very painful cramps, bloating, body aches, and body consequences that leave me on the couch for four to seven days at a time. I am often emotional, in deep pain, and in a great amount of discomfort. I can't wear much of the clothing that I usually wear to construct and feel comfortable in my gender, like chest binders, so I don't often leave the house. I can't exercise, feel so unsexy and undesirous, and often am miserable to be around as a friend or lover.

There are a variety of things that can cause heavy bleeding and periods. Polycystic ovary syndrome (PCOS) and endometriosis are common causes, for example. I've been tested for many of these things and everything always checked out healthy.

When I mentioned painful periods to my nurse practitioners during annual exams over the years, they responded immediately with, "Birth control pills would alleviate that." When I told them I'm genderqueer and identify as transmasculine and asked what estrogen would do to my system, they almost always said they had no idea, but that taking estrogen was the only option. Have I tried taking hot baths, they would ask, or taking some ibuprofen?

Cue my incredulous face.

Fuck yes, I have tried ibuprofen. Actually, my drug of choice is naproxen (Aleve), but I started getting nervous about how bad it is for me when two nurse friends of mine described how excessive use (and oh yes, I used it excessively) would make your stomach bleed. So maybe, I thought, I should seek other treatment.

And also, Nurse: How can you not know what the hormones will do to my body? You're the one recommending them, yet you don't know or understand the consequences?

(Nobody really knows how hormones work, I know now. But none of my doctors were transparent about this.)

And how can you not have any other options for heavy bleeding than to flatten out my natural hormonal cycle with pills? Could there be something wrong underneath the surface that is causing this intense cycle? What could be wrong? Could we perhaps treat that instead?

It is not news to me that the medical industry does not take "women's issues" like heavy, painful periods seriously. The female practitioners I saw clearly did not have experience with it themselves, or I'm pretty sure they would have a) treated it and b) had more options. Not that that's a surprise—my undergraduate degree in women's and gender studies certainly included plenty of health classes that discussed the othering of women and women's bodies at length. But this felt different: This was *my* body.

I reached a breaking point one month, on day two of my bleeding period, when I cried in the car as my partner went to the hour-long workout we had planned together. In one of the moments when the pain lifted, and then later to my partner over breakfast, I vowed: I have to do something, anything. I cannot live like this anymore. There have to be options. Even estrogen.

I started treatment with a Chinese herbalist practitioner. I took an assortment of teas and herbs, coming in multiple times a month for acupuncture and assessments. And I started doing research on hormonal birth control options for trans men—not because I identify as male, but because there must be options that don't interfere with taking testosterone and transitioning. What I found—mostly on Tumblr and Livejournal and personal blogs—were trans men describing what they knew about how hormones work, which birth control options helped their heavy periods, and which didn't affect their doses of testosterone.

Let me stress this point: I did my own research. The doctors did not help. The information I found was from personal sources telling their own stories and sharing what they found. I don't love the idea of crowdsourcing my own health and wellness, getting solutions to medical problems on Tumblr, but with a body that's an unknown in the medical system, what else was I supposed to do?

I feel naïve for trusting the medical system over my own body for so long.

The herbs helped with pain but not with the underlying issues, so I sought a more sustainable solution. Not long after my declaration, the health care act in the US passed. I qualified for insurance through Obamacare and started going to my local trans-friendly clinic, assuming that they would know about hormones. I made an appointment, armed with the research that I'd done and a proposal for a solution—the Mirena IUD, which is progesterone-based and wouldn't add more estrogen to my system.

It was a relief to go somewhere where queer and trans bodies were valued. They had a special place on their intake form for my preferred name, and they used it when calling me in for my appointment. They asked about pronouns; they didn't use gendered language when referring to my body. It was such a relief, and something in me relaxed that I didn't even know I was holding.

But they still didn't always know how to help, and they still didn't always trust that I was the expert of my own body.

I wrote about my experiences online and I declared that my intention was to pursue the Mirena, which seemed like my best bet. An entirely new conversation opened up from that piece of writing. People asked all kinds of useful questions, and suggested ideas or things that had helped them. A lot of trans and genderqueer folks weighed in and commiserated with the experience of being overlooked, ignored, or not taken seriously by the health care system. Many shared their experience with the Mirena—some good, some terrible. And eventually, a practitioner out of Canada, Rose Yewchuk, who used the Justisse method, contacted me and I began working with her.

"Give Justisse six months," Rose said. Adding IUD hormones into my system could solve the superficial issue of my heavy periods, but it wouldn't tell me what was going on behind that. Justisse, on the other hand, assessed the whole body and the entire system, and could offer insights about what was throwing my cycle off in the first place.

Justisse is a cycle-charting method where you keep track of your cervical mucus and basal body temperature in order to show patterns and irregularities in your cycle based on those data points. Rose suggested supplements based on the charts she read, and I felt like they made a difference. Finally, I was getting somewhere! Plus, she's trans-friendly, genderqueer-aware, and very willing to ask questions and learn more about how my body works. She trusts my own authority on my gender and my health. She believes I know better than she does, but that she has a variety of knowledge that might help with what I'm going through. She uses my pronouns. It was such a relief to work with someone where I no longer got called "miss" and "lady" all the time.

After a few months of charting, I went back to my doctor to have some new tests taken, and still: nothing. No clear answers about what was causing this difficulty. I did see some progress—the supplements were clearly doing something good, and my pain was lessening. But my charts were still a little off, and the pain was still high.

I kept up with it, but felt I'd plateaued. I bought yet more supplements and spent yet more money on expensive bottles of herbs and remedies, and my daily pill box became too full to hold them all. That was when I started learning about muscle testing, a way to tell whether something is resonating with the body, something I'd only previously done in spiritual practice.

The embodiment practices I've done for my own personal growth over the years have deepened into a philosophical, scientific, and spiritual system to which I am devoted. What started as a desire to have more knowledge of my and others' erotic bodies became a place to explore deep pleasure, release trauma, uncover truths, and know myself. A significant piece of my practice is about my own body, taking care of it, being aware of what is unconscious, and doing more of what feeds and nourishes me well. Practices such as movement, meditation, rest, and detoxification are foundational. In conjunction with this experience of failure in the western medical system, I became more and more convinced that maintaining, monitoring, and enhancing my own health and well-being is a key part of my spiritual practice.

How could I have put my own well-being in the hands of doctors for so long? Doctors who looked at tests and told me my body was fine, even when I was sitting right there telling them that my body was saying otherwise. Doctors who called me "miss" and "ma'am" and "lady." Doctors who had no idea how their prescriptions would interact with my body, but told me that it was my only option. And doctors who told me my health problems would all be fixed if I lost weight. (Hello, can we talk about fatphobia for a minute? While it has only been a minor thread in this whole experience for me, I know it is a major one for others, and the moments I've felt it have been intense and real.)

No wonder I didn't trust them. No wonder I didn't get the help I needed. I felt failed by the health care system.

I know the health care system fails many, many people and, comparatively, I am very privileged to have been able to both afford and access the care that I have been pursuing. But I do want to keep this in perspective—I still feel like the system failed me.

I didn't really know what was going on with my body until I finally dug deep enough, with four different practitioners helping me to pursue what was going on with my body, and I sent away for a blood test from the internet.

After Rose and I had gone through many of the possible options, the next thing to investigate was some sort of food allergy, so I had an IgG allergy blood test done. When the test came back, most of the foods were within very normal ranges, and only one section was off the charts: candida. The results finally, finally, showed an answer for what was going on with my body. But it might still be covering up something else going on underneath, Rose warned me. Candida is a treatable, common thing that can have a huge effect on one's body. So the aim was to get this taken care of, and then keep finding out more.

I brought this information to my primary care practitioner, who knew almost nothing about it—it's not an issue that western medicine acknowledges or treats. My herbalist seemed a bit flippant about it. The Facebook group of those who suffer from it is extraordinarily dramatic, with members often making bold internet click-bait headline declarations of how they are going to "die if these symptoms continue for one more day!!"

But for me, the diagnosis is a hard-won victory of knowing and trusting my own body. It took climbing over transphobia and cissexism to get here. It took undoing my own internalized hierarchical systems of trusting western medicine doctors and institutions to tell me what was wrong with my body. It took advocating for myself and my own knowledge of my body when I came up against a system that didn't understand me or, I felt, even try to understand me.

My relationships with my body and with the health care system in the US are forever changed by this experience. I am pickier about practitioners that I trust and more of an active participant in my own health. I consider my health part of my spiritual practice, everything from herbs to food to experiences at the doctor to self-care. I trust my own genderqueerness and body sensitivity as part of my gift, and am listening even louder now to my own inner knowing.

It's not over or complete—I have to re-listen and re-learn frequently.

And who knows what will be next, after I get the candida levels back to average. But I trust that I can do it now, that I have better tools in my belt, and that I won't let the system tell me what is or is not true for me again.

If there is a collective noun for my people, it could be a stubborn. Never mess with a stubborn of queers.

OUR CAREGIVING, OURSELVES

Kelli Dunham

It's rare that Seriously Observant Religious People and Seriously Culturally Queer People find themselves on the same side of any argument, let alone co-conspirators against a common authority figure.

But when my partner Cheryl was dying of pulmonary complications from chemo that was supposed to cure her Hodgkin's lymphoma, our large, extremely unorthodox queer family shared many hours in ICU waiting rooms with equally large extended Orthodox Jewish families. We were as friendly as we could be across hard tile and the smell of hospital antiseptic and the fear of death and countless unspoken assumptions.

Members of the various caregiving teams, including me, wedged ourselves into small physical spaces and into the cracks of permission we had to be physically present for our family members who were fighting for their lives. The rule that established maximum number of visitors (two during the day, one at night) in the ICU made sense; the patient rooms were crammed with very ill people and the sensitive and expensive equipment keeping them alive.

However, while we were careful only to have at most two folks at Cheryl's bedside at a time, the sheer number of people who were rotating through seemed to alarm the staff. They would establish temporary and arbitrary rules that had no discernible purpose except for discouraging this rotation. For example, they'd decide that only one person was allowed to be present at a patient's bedside between eleven p.m. and seven a.m. By this they didn't mean one person at a time; this would have made sense based on the Small Spaces/Sick Patient argument. Instead, their one-person rule meant that just one specific individual could be with a patient in that eight-hour period, no swap-outs allowed.

Patients who had mostly small families of the nuclear biological variety were not affected by the no swap-out rule since there was no one waiting to take over. But for those of us working in teams as family or large families as teams, it messed up our whole system.

But it also did nothing to discourage us. The surest way to get a bunch of queers to do anything is to make a rule nonsensically forbidding us from doing it. If there is a collective noun for my people, it could be a stubborn. Never mess with a stubborn of queers.

A stubborn of queers will not leave their dying friend because someone in charge tells them to. And as for me, the first night I spent away from Cheryl in her ultimately almost three-month hospitalization, she texted me at three a.m.: "I'm scared and alone and I can't breathe." One text like that was 100 percent more than I could handle. After that I camped out at the hospital like I was paying rent.

One night early during Cheryl's first stint in the ICU, I had spent four hours with my larger-than-average ass stuffed into the smaller-than-average visitor chairs in the waiting room. I chatted with my close friend Zed, who was there to support Cheryl and me. Zed was chilly, so I offered them my blue tattered sweatshirt. When Zed stretched in the doorway of the waiting room, a nurse gestured to them.

"Hurry up. Are you coming back in or not?"

Zed looked at me as I shook with suppressed laughter and crouched down into my chair. Because Zed was wearing my sweatshirt, the nurse thought they were me. Aside from both being queers on the trans-masculine spectrum—and now, being seen in the same hoodie—we looked nothing alike. I winked and Zed trotted into Cheryl's ICU room to finish out the night shift.

I looked over at one of the Orthodox men curled up in the corner and shot him a covert signal about what had just transpired by raising an eyebrow. Message received, he quickly sent a text message to his cousin visiting their loved one, and when his cousin exited the ICU, they conducted a similar exchange with an overcoat.

The Super Gay Sweatshirt and the Orthodox Overcoat made numerous appearances that spring and summer. At the time I'd been a practicing registered nurse for more than fifteen years so I had more than the occasional guilt pang about deceiving the exhausted and overworked hospital staff. At the same time, the fact that the ongoing rotations enabled by our subterfuge didn't cause any actual problems reinforced how silly the hospital rules were in the first place.

I would be very surprised if the hospital staff were motivated by homophobia in their lack of enthusiasm for our Big Fat Queer Caregiving Group. In fact, they went out of their way to include me as the partner in all things relating to Cheryl. The social worker on the palliative care team even took the initiative to make multiple copies of our health care proxy paperwork so it could be easily found in Cheryl's chart and so I could also carry a copy with me.

The staff got the partner part. What they didn't get was who the hell all those other people were. From their vantage point, the parade of family members and friends through the hospital represented potential chaos.

The problem was not that staff had this vantage point; families and friends can sometimes exhaust patients with their well-meaning attention.

The problem was that staff didn't base their judgment on the reality of the relationship between Cheryl, me, and our queer family. If staff had looked closer—and perhaps even inquired directly with Cheryl—they would have understood that no one from our queer family was distracting me from taking care of Cheryl. On the contrary, their involvement made it possible for me to do so.

I moved into the hospital when Cheryl was admitted and slept there every night except one. When Cheryl was well enough to be in a regular room for a time, I brought in a sleeping bag, mattress pad, pillow, and teddy bear and made a cozy bed on the radiator beside her. This would have been logistically unmanageable without our "chaotic" queer family. Every time I was hungry, a hamburger would magically appear in my right hand and a Diet Mountain Dew in my left. Every so often, a fresh set of clothes would be draped across my arm with the gentle suggestion, "I can sit with Cheryl for a bit, go grab a shower."

Since Cheryl's death, I've been involved with many groups of queers organizing caregiving teams, and they often run into institutional resistance caused by a restrictive model that insists that family begins and ends with whomever is deemed the primary partner.

This is sad for the person needing care and their caregiving team, but there is a loss to the greater community as well. We know that isolated experiences of caregiving are a devastating blow to the physical, emotional, and financial health of a solitary caregiver. And we know that because of the aging population of the Baby Boomers, we are headed toward a family caregiving crisis of unrivaled proportions.

Not every queer person comes equipped with the kind of team that Cheryl had. But our group caregiving skills—necessitated by isolation from biological family and refined in the furnace of the AIDS crisis—are a well-documented strength of our community. Instead of turning an exceptional strength into a pesky problem that needs to be fixed, health care providers might embrace the model of group caregiving and then perhaps even teach subsequent families about how to build a team of caregivers based on what they've learned from us. Hospital staff should not mistake our passion for stridency: expanding the definition of who and what makes a family may stretch the limits of their emotional understanding, but it has been literally lifesaving for us.

QUEER IN COMMON COUNTRY

Kara Sievewright

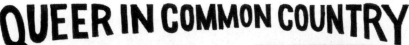

QUEER IN COMMON COUNTRY

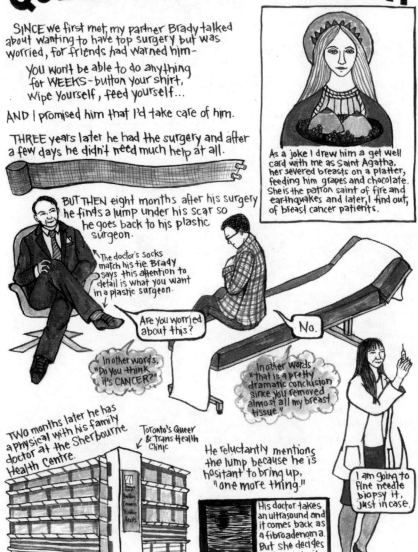

SINCE we first met, my partner Brady talked about wanting to have top surgery but was worried, for friends had warned him—

YOU won't be able to do anything for WEEKS—button your shirt, wipe yourself, feed yourself...

AND I promised him that I'd take care of him.

THREE years later he had the surgery and after a few days he didn't need much help at all.

As a joke I drew him a get well card with me as Saint Agatha, her severed breasts on a platter, feeding him grapes and chocolate. She is the patron saint of fire and earthquakes and later, I find out, of breast cancer patients.

BUT THEN eight months after his surgery he finds a lump under his scar so he goes back to his plastic surgeon.

The doctor's socks match his tie. Brady says this attention to detail is what you want in a plastic surgeon.

Are you worried about this?

No.

In other words, "Do you think it's CANCER?"

In other words, "that is a pretty dramatic conclusion since you removed almost all my breast tissue."

TWO months later he has a physical with his family doctor at the Sherbourne Health Centre.

Toronto's Queer & Trans Health Clinic

He reluctantly mentions the lump because he is hesitant to bring up, "one more thing."

His doctor takes an ultrasound and it comes back as a fibroadenoma. But she decides to look into it further.

I am going to fine needle biopsy it, just in case.

TWO WEEKS later, he goes back to her office for the results. I don't go because we know it is nothing, how could it be anything, the odds are against it and there is no way that he is not on the favourable side, on the side against the possibility of it being anything.

Many people have this story...

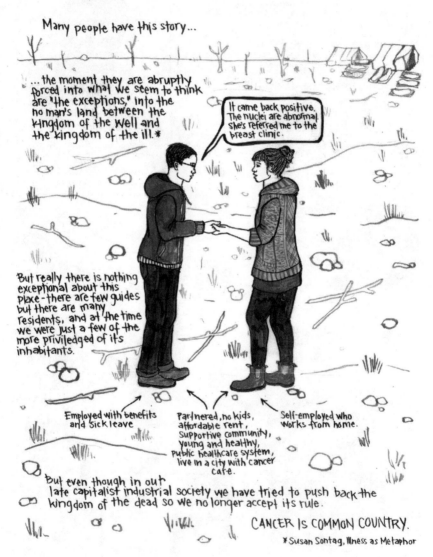

...the moment they are abruptly forced into what we seem to think are "the exceptions," into the no man's land between the kingdom of the well and the kingdom of the ill.*

It came back positive. The nuclei are abnormal. She's refered me to the breast clinic.

But really there is nothing exceptional about this place - there are few guides but there are many residents, and at the time we were just a few of the more priviledged of its inhabitants.

Employed with benefits and sick leave

Partnered, no kids, affordable rent, supportive community, young and healthy, public healthcare system, live in a city with cancer care.

Self-employed who works from home.

But even though in our late capitalist industrial society we have tried to push back the kingdom of the dead so we no longer accept its rule.

CANCER IS COMMON COUNTRY.

* Susan Sontag, Illness as Metaphor

A WEEK LATER the breast clinic calls but when we go to the appointment two weeks later they tell us that they rebooked it and to come back in another two weeks.

All that spring, I remember, in that time between appointments I would walk to my studio with thoughts, worries, fears, panic, decisions multiplying high above me like cumulonimbus clouds.

What if it's cancer?

What if he dies?

What if he has to have chemo?

Will we be able to move back to the west coast like we planned?

What if he dies?

What about all those who have died from breast cancer... mothers, aunts, grandmothers, Kathy Acker, Audre Lorde, Lhasa...

Maybe it is nothing, it is probably nothing.

If we could just create plans and possibilities, if we could only be on the otherside of knowing.

Meanwhile in his body cells are dividing, multiplying.

Later I tell my roommate and her girlfriend, both nurses, that the doctors must not think that Brady's case is that urgent because they have been making us wait so long for appointments.
They look at each other and scoff with the knowledge of insiders. "I wouldn't take it to mean that at all," they say.

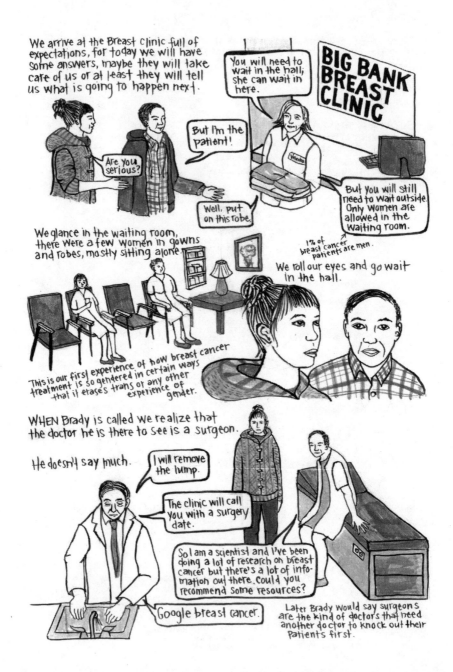

We arrive at the Breast Clinic full of expectations, for today we will have some answers, maybe they will take care of us or at least they will tell us what is going to happen next.

Are you serious?

But I'm the patient!

Well, put on this robe.

You will need to wait in the hall; she can wait in here.

BIG BANK BREAST CLINIC

But you will still need to wait outside. Only women are allowed in the waiting room.

We glance in the waiting room, there were a few women in gowns and robes, mostly sitting alone.

1% of breast cancer patients are men.

We roll our eyes and go wait in the hall.

This is our first experience of how breast cancer treatment is so gendered in certain ways that it erases trans or any other experience of gender.

WHEN Brady is called we realize that the doctor he is there to see is a surgeon.

He doesn't say much.

I will remove the lump.

The clinic will call you with a surgery date.

So I am a scientist and I've been doing a lot of research on breast cancer but there's a lot of information out there. Could you recommend some resources?

Google breast cancer.

Later Brady would say surgeons are the kind of doctors that need another doctor to knock out their patients first.

92

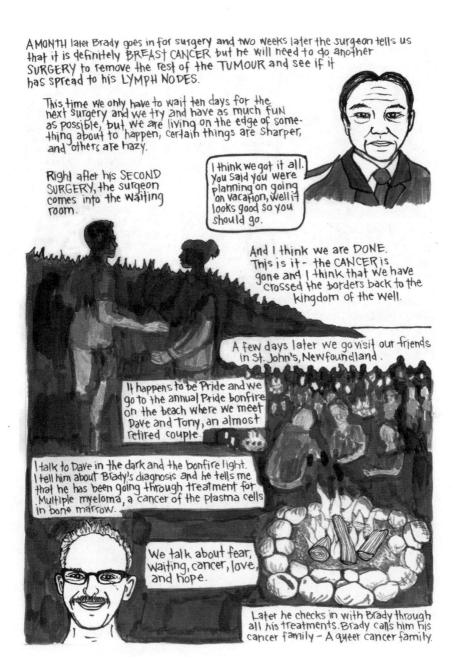

A MONTH later Brady goes in for surgery and two weeks later the surgeon tells us that it is definitely BREAST CANCER but he will need to do another SURGERY to remove the rest of the TUMOUR and see if it has spread to his LYMPH NODES.

This time we only have to wait ten days for the next surgery and we try and have as much fun as possible, but we are living on the edge of something about to happen, certain things are sharper, and others are hazy.

Right after his SECOND SURGERY, the surgeon comes into the waiting room.

I think we got it all. You said you were planning on going on vacation, well it looks good so you should go.

And I think we are DONE. This is it - the CANCER is gone and I think that we have crossed the borders back to the kingdom of the well.

A few days later we go visit our friends in St. John's, Newfoundland.

It happens to be Pride and we go to the annual Pride bonfire on the beach where we meet Dave and Tony, an almost retired couple.

I talk to Dave in the dark and the bonfire light. I tell him about Brady's diagnosis and he tells me that he has been going through treatment for Multiple myeloma, a cancer of the plasma cells in bone marrow.

We talk about fear, waiting, cancer, love, and hope.

Later he checks in with Brady through all his treatments. Brady calls him his cancer family – A queer cancer family.

93

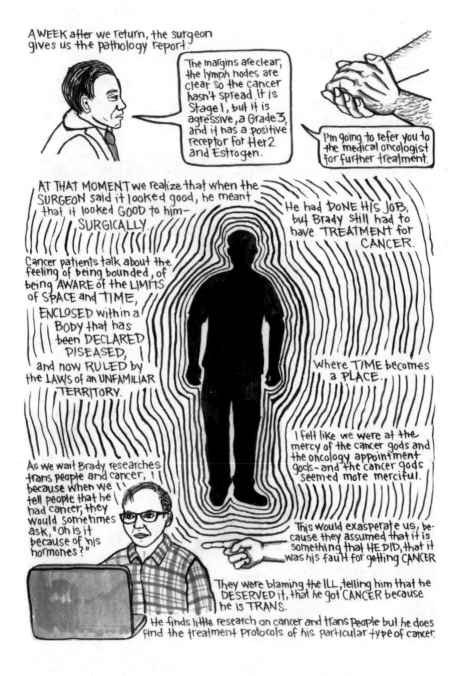

A WEEK after we return, the surgeon gives us the pathology report.

The margins are clear, the lymph nodes are clear so the cancer hasn't spread. It is Stage 1, but it is aggressive, a Grade 3, and it has a positive receptor for Her 2 and Estrogen.

I'm going to refer you to the medical oncologist for further treatment.

AT THAT MOMENT we realize that when the SURGEON said it looked good, he meant that it looked GOOD to him— SURGICALLY.

He had DONE HIS JOB, but Brady still had to have TREATMENT for CANCER.

Cancer patients talk about the feeling of being bounded, of being AWARE of the LIMITS of SPACE and TIME, ENCLOSED within a BODY that has been DECLARED DISEASED, and now RULED by the LAWS of an UNFAMILIAR TERRITORY.

Where TIME becomes a PLACE.

As we wait Brady researches trans people and cancer, because when we tell people that he had cancer, they would sometimes ask, "Oh is it because of his hormones?"

I felt like we were at the mercy of the cancer gods and the oncology appointment gods—and the cancer gods seemed more merciful.

This would exasperate us, because they assumed that it is something that HE DID, that it was his fault for getting CANCER

They were blaming the ILL, telling him that he DESERVED it, that he got CANCER because he is TRANS.

He finds little research on cancer and trans people but he does find the treatment protocols of his particular type of cancer.

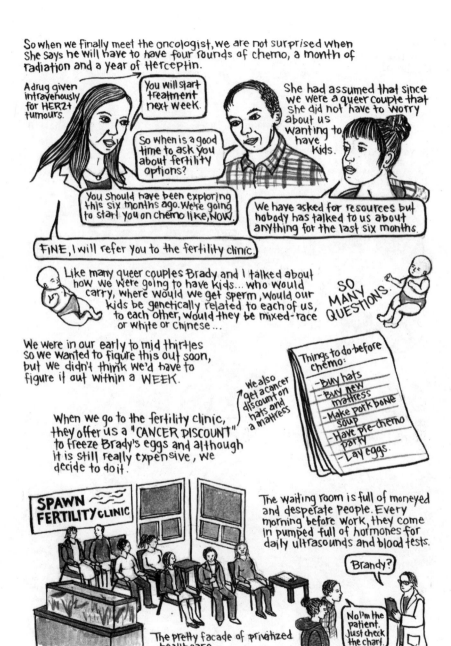

So when we finally meet the oncologist, we are not surprised when she says he will have to have four rounds of chemo, a month of radiation and a year of Herceptin.

A drug given intravenously for HER2+ tumours.

You will start treatment next week.

So when is a good time to ask you about fertility options?

She had assumed that since we were a queer couple that she did not have to worry about us wanting to have kids.

You should have been exploring this six months ago. We're going to start you on chemo like, NOW.

We have asked for resources but nobody has talked to us about anything for the last six months.

FINE, I will refer you to the fertility clinic.

Like many queer couples Brady and I talked about how we were going to have kids... who would carry, where would we get sperm, would our kids be genetically related to each of us, to each other, would they be mixed-race or white or Chinese...

SO MANY QUESTIONS.

We were in our early to mid thirties so we wanted to figure this out soon, but we didn't think we'd have to figure it out within a WEEK.

When we go to the fertility clinic, they offer us a "CANCER DISCOUNT" to freeze Brady's eggs and although it is still really expensive, we decide to do it.

We also get a cancer discount on hats and a mattress

Things to do before chemo:
- Buy hats
- Buy new mattress
- Make pork bone soup
- Have pre-chemo party
- Lay eggs.

SPAWN FERTILITY CLINIC

The waiting room is full of moneyed and desperate people. Every morning before work, they come in pumped full of hormones for daily ultrasounds and blood tests.

Brandy?

No, I'm the patient. Just check the chart.

The pretty facade of privatized healthcare.

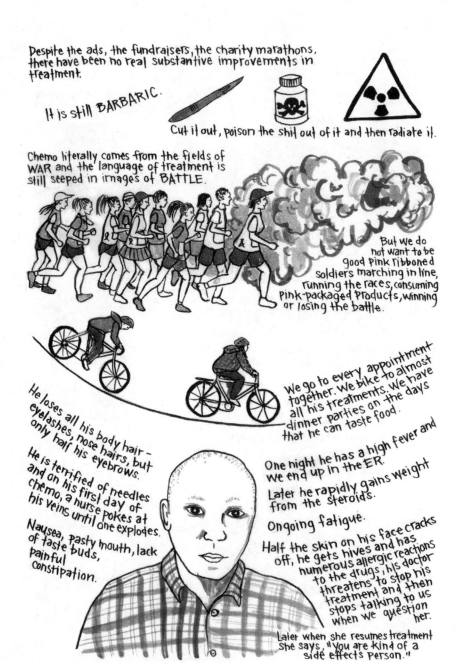

Despite the ads, the fundraisers, the charity marathons, there have been no real substantive improvements in treatment.

It is still BARBARIC.

Cut it out, poison the shit out of it and then radiate it.

Chemo literally comes from the fields of WAR and the language of treatment is still steeped in images of BATTLE.

But we do not want to be good pink ribboned soldiers marching in line, running the races, consuming pink-packaged products, winning or losing the battle.

We go to every appointment together. We bike to almost all his treatments. We have dinner parties on the days that he can taste food.

He loses all his body hair – eyelashes, nose hairs, but only half his eyebrows.

He is terrified of needles and on his first day of chemo, a nurse pokes at his veins until one explodes.

Nausea, pasty mouth, lack of taste buds, painful constipation.

One night he has a high fever and we end up in the ER.

Later he rapidly gains weight from the steroids.

Ongoing fatigue.

Half the skin on his face cracks off, he gets hives and has numerous allergic reactions to the drugs, his doctor threatens to stop his treatment and then stops talking to us when we question her.

Later when she resumes treatment she says, "You are kind of a side effects person."

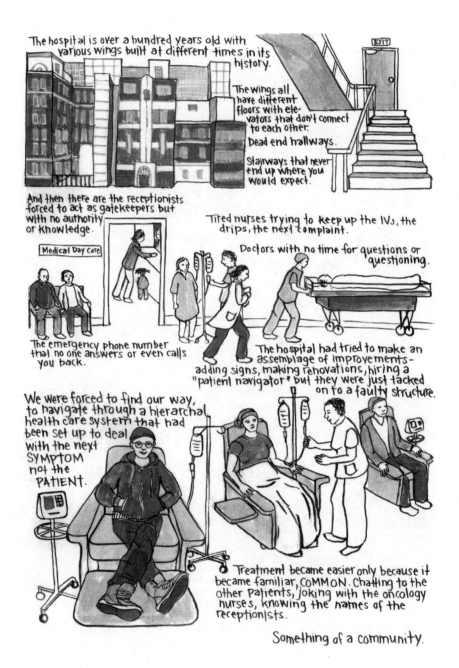

The hospital is over a hundred years old with various wings built at different times in its history.

The wings all have different floors with elevators that don't connect to each other.

Dead end hallways.

Stairways that never end up where you would expect.

EXIT

And then there are the receptionists forced to act as gatekeepers but with no authority or knowledge.

Medical Day Care

Tired nurses trying to keep up the IVs, the drips, the next complaint.

Doctors with no time for questions or questioning.

The emergency phone number that no one answers or even calls you back.

The hospital had tried to make an assemblage of improvements—adding signs, making renovations, hiring a "patient navigator" but they were just tacked on to a faulty structure.

We were forced to find our way, to navigate through a hierarchal health care system that had been set up to deal with the next SYMPTOM not the PATIENT.

Treatment became easier only because it became familiar, COMMON. Chatting to the other patients, joking with the oncology nurses, knowing the names of the receptionists.

Something of a community.

97

These small communities – not SOLID or ENCLOSED as to be disappointing or exclusive.

Just being with and getting through.

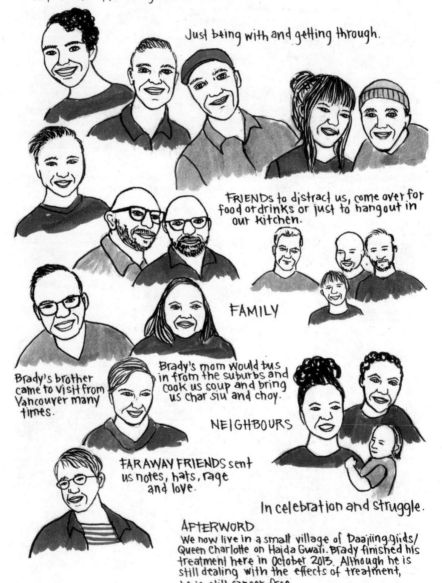

FRIENDS to distract us, come over for food or drinks or just to hangout in our kitchen.

FAMILY

Brady's brother came to visit from Vancouver many times.

Brady's mom would bus in from the suburbs and cook us soup and bring us char siu and choy.

NEIGHBOURS

FARAWAY FRIENDS sent us notes, hats, rage and love.

In celebration and struggle.

AFTERWORD
We now live in a small village of Daajiing.giids/ Queen Charlotte on Haida Gwaii. Brady finished his treatment here in October 2013. Although he is still dealing with the effects of treatment, he is still cancer free.

Whether I knew it or not, at the time, I was the "other." I consider this to be one of life's ironies, an Indigenous person feeling alien in their own land.

NIRKwUSCIN

Chase Willier

In memory of my adopted father, Glen Douglas, whose voice still echoes.

As someone who is both older and supposedly wiser, I consider myself blessed to have come from a culture where my elders acknowledged the two-spirit aspects of my identity, both as a lesbian and now, years later, as a transman. Like so many aboriginal people in Canada and a child of the Sixties Scoop, when First Nations children were "scooped" from their families and placed in foster homes or adopted, I struggled with a myriad of losses, and had no idea how deeply they had affected me. That's the hangover of colonization, a toxic cocktail of negative emotions, all swirling around with nowhere to go. I could feel a deep sense of frustration inside, but it took a while before I began to have words for it, and even longer to finally express my hurt, anger, and grief. Had it not been for my elders, who traditionally adopted me into the Syilx Nation at a very critical time in my life, my outcome would have been entirely different. At a gathering on Westbank First Nation, Glen Douglas embraced me in a blanket, took me in as his own, and he and his wife Lesley gave me the nurturing, guidance, and teachings I so desperately needed. Those early experiences gave me a compass, helping me sail through many a storm in a journey that has not only been a challenge, but has also held more than a few unexpected surprises.

"Culture is Healing," or at least that's what Round Lake Alcohol and

Drug Treatment Centre's logo said when I started volunteering for the women's sweat lodge every Tuesday. That was over thirty years ago, and ceremony and ritual are still a central part of my wellness. Other modalities, like psychotherapy and bodywork, have also played an important role. It wasn't always the case, as it took several years to be able to get any real results using the health care system. My first forays into counselling really lacked in meeting my needs. I have to preface this by saying that as a Royal Canadian Mounted Police (RCMP) officer at the time, I had excellent health care coverage and seeking out a force-approved psychologist wasn't an issue. The problem was that the practitioners I encountered either had little experience working with First Nations peoples, or their beliefs around wellness didn't seem to align with mine. It was evident that cultural competencies weren't on the radar screen during my initial explorations, so I stumbled my way through, never establishing a meaningful connection. An indigenous therapist wasn't available to me, either because they weren't on the approved list, or because they were not accessible in my area. Not only was I in the closet, a lesbian working in uniform as an RCMP officer in the 1980s, but I was also a First Nations woman. I was an anomaly, much like today, being transgendered. I couldn't help but feel isolated, and engaging with the health care system amplified the discomfort. Whether I knew it or not, at the time I was the "other." I consider this to be one of life's ironies, an Indigenous person feeling alien in their own land.

Mental health was a term that seemed innocuous enough, but it was still suspect. It didn't fit into my worldview around holistic healing and the interconnectedness of the physical, emotional, mental, and spiritual. I floundered around with a general lack of trust, wasting not only my time but the practitioners', where the hours spent were lost following breadcrumbs through a maze of roads that never led anywhere. The many interruptions that came along, caused by my having to answer the inquiring minds wanting or needing to be educated on my time were not helpful towards establishing confidence. Granted, said minds were learning about First Nations, but ... I chalked it up to my somewhat unique situation and made allowances for it, something I later realized I had become conditioned to do. And although my practitioners were well meaning, their attempts felt like token gestures. One needs to remember that the Sixties Scoop had its fair share of do-gooders and social workers who honestly thought they were acting in the best interests of the child. These actions along with other atrocities including Indian residential schools are a part of my collective history of colonization. Suffice to say that it was some time before any real results were gleaned. I had yet to experience cultural safety.

When I reflect back upon my many interactions with mental health professionals, one of the things that astonishes me is the absence of the conversation around post-traumatic stress disorder (PTSD). Surely, as an RCMP officer, this was a possibility and, certainly with my history, a logical conclusion. While posted in the Okanagan, with family, community, and support systems that included strong cultural ties, I excelled at work. However, the sense of dread, which I had become quite adept at avoiding, was triggered by a transfer to the Sechelt Detachment in the spring of 1990. I was placed on "stress leave," and couldn't understand what was going on with my body. The harder I pushed myself, the worse it got. The diagnosis was "reactive depression" to the transfer, which would partially explain what was happening. Yet I recalled Glen talking about his PTSD on many occasions (he was a highly decorated veteran, having served in the US military during three wars), and I often wondered about myself. But he also spoke about how colonization affected our people, particularly around his being a survivor of Indian residential schools. I had no idea as to how this would affect me—after all, I didn't go to any residential schools.

It wasn't until a decade later, while working with a lesbian clinical counsellor, that I discovered a practitioner who actually used the "C" word. Finally, I was being acknowledged as someone who came from a history of trauma and loss, resulting from colonization. I also began to see how oppression wasn't just a First Nations experience for me. There were other intersections at play, and I could now acknowledge other aspects of self which, surprisingly, brought up the same feelings. Finding the vibrant gay community in Vancouver really helped me shed the layer of shame that had kept me isolated for so long. It honestly surprised me, the sense of true freedom and happiness just being at ease with self and finding community. My elders were accepting of my two-spirit identity, and Glen told me a story of an Okanagan woman who was also two spirit and was a highly revered war chief. I couldn't help but feel even more connected to culture.

His elder, in Nespelum, Washington, still remembered a time before contact, when not only being a woman, but gender identity and expression were healthy and thriving. Today, our communities are still recovering from the "isms" and "obias" introduced with colonization and, far too often, two-spirit/transgendered people are the target of hatred. Sadly, it comes from both worlds, not just on reserve or in small communities, but also when two-spirit/transfolk escape to the city to find community only to once again encounter racism, trans/homophobia, and other challenges. I can't help but think of spawning salmon swimming upstream, fighting to reach a goal that may be unattainable.

Transitioning reminds me of my struggles growing up. The feeling of vulnerability and the potential for violence are similar, only this time it's my gender or lack thereof, not race, that is the issue for many around me. And, although I have learned to temper my hypervigilance, which is part of my PTSD, I remain acutely aware of my surroundings. The classic hallmark stares I get due to my lack of conforming to the gender binary will be with me until my body fully transitions. However, it is the more subtle assaults that are difficult to see coming, and that often leave me in doubt. The change in attitude of the once-friendly, conversational ultrasound therapist who suddenly shifts to cold and mute is suspect. Other, more hurtful actions conducted in public carry the same harsh blows as racism inflicts. I refer to this as the deer-in-the-headlights phenomenon. Somehow, I'm always stunned and unprepared, rarely able to respond, because I feel like I've been kicked in the chest. The internalized anger at myself for not immediately challenging the incident is exacerbated since I'm temporarily winded and without words. The pain is deep and debilitating. There resides a level of frustration and rawness that exists below the surface that only my brothers and sisters know. It keeps the "other" isolated, questioning their sanity and self-worth. It would explain the statistics around suicide for First Nations people, for transfolk, and so many others who are marginalized; after a lifetime of constant reinjury or aggravation, a person's ability to withstand these assaults is whittled away.

Sometimes, that's when they enter the health care system. They may be desperately in need of help, but are unwilling or resistant, especially if experience has shown them that they will be judged, or worse. Often, they enter the system as a last resort, the cost of not trying one last, fatal time.

Some thirty years later, as a retired RCMP officer full of confidence and life experience, I'm reminded of how deep those wounds are the moment I ask for help. The role of shame is a powerful and a pervasive presence, even today. Advocating for self, having a voice and being able to use it, has not been an easy lesson. Asserting myself and confronting an issue around my health care is probably one of the most accurate measures of my self-worth. One of my most difficult experiences in health care occurred at the UBC Operational Stress Injury Clinic when I was first assessed and sought treatment for my PTSD. I was already experiencing considerable anxiety which I tried to control with avoidance behaviours (something I'd become extremely adept at doing). So, when I sensed judgment from the practitioner early on, I began to stress over our sessions rather than the actual trauma work itself, and things began to unravel. Somehow I felt in the wrong, and full of self-doubt.

Was it my trans identity? Was it race? I tried not to project. Whatever it was, something was undermining our sessions. I needed to advocate for self, address the problem, and request another counsellor. My resistance to rocking the boat and my fear around exacerbating the situation were grounded in previous experiences. Prior conflicts usually proved that I wasn't the one in power, and that I would get hurt. The idea of putting oneself at further risk goes against anyone's nature.

Fortunately, this issue was managed efficiently, and within a short period of time, I was assigned a new practitioner, Dr. Mollie Bates. Surprisingly, things moved along quickly and trust was established early on, since the presence of respect, empathy, and non-judgement in the room was palpable. I suspected that this practitioner understood that people coming from a long history with oppression have their own mechanisms and tools they use to survive. I am no different. Not only is my history with colonization complex, but it's also cumulative in nature, specifically around trauma. Grief and loss are not the same as someone coming from a nuclear family where they may not have lost a family member until they were an adult nor suffered disconnection from community, language, or culture as a result of government policies. My faith and trust in a counsellor who is capable of discussing privilege as it relates to oppression is well placed. I know I'm in good hands, and I also know the person who sits across from me not only has done her own work, but has taken responsibility for it. I've never had to educate my practitioner on competencies around my identities, nor is it my responsibility anymore. I have expectations around respect, cultural competencies, and a shared learning environment.

Active listening skills are a part of that since it's how I know if someone is genuine or not. In general, law enforcement personnel interrupt someone speaking every seven to nine seconds. Quick assessment is required under certain conditions, particularly for emergency responders, so this practice is understandable—within the workplace.

However, certain practices that work under specific conditions do not carry over to the "other." And more often than not, two cultures (whether they be First Nations, queer/trans, and yes, even policing and health care) usually come into conflict. There must be a mindfulness around listening and respect which is just the beginning of the relationship.

Creating safe space requires hard work. And if there's anything I know for a fact, it's that safety is absolutely essential to my wellness. As my identities are acknowledged and given a voice, only then can I move into a space beyond survival mode. In a way it reminds me of ceremony where certain conditions have to be carefully prepared in order for spirit to come: it's the respectful tones, the welcoming, the coming together in a way that honours the other.

His office felt like a safe space where I was respected for who I was. He saw me as
a unique individual with agency and self-determination, and that felt good.

A JOURNEY
TOWARDS SAFETY

Ahmed Danny Ramadan

She tells me that controlling my social anxiety is as easy as controlling the way I breathe. I need to inhale for four counts, hold it in for two, then release the air in six calming, relaxing counts, and repeat until I feel calmer. Four-Two-Six: like a football game strategy, easy to remember, simple to practice. But I don't believe her.

What is this counsellor talking about and why does she want to control my breathing! I start to give excuses to refuse anything she says. I completely lose trust in her and her work, and I talk myself into "rebelling" against this system that I found myself in.

My counsellor, a white woman in her late forties, tried to talk me into calming down, tried to guide me through meditation techniques, and to talk to me about stress levels. She spoke an alien language. I detested my visits to her; they felt like a burden. Her words as she guided me through my issues felt enforced and belittling. Her voice felt like scratches on the side of my brain.

She doesn't understand who I am; she will never know or experience the things I know. I feel more and more disconnected from the new community that I thought would be my sanctuary.

I didn't realize it back then, but when I arrived in Canada, I was very tired. I was tired after being a gay Syrian refugee in Lebanon for two years, working hard on meeting the very basics of life needs: water to drink, food to eat, shelter to provide warmth, and dignified work. There was only one that I didn't require: physical safety. Feeling safe was not an issue for me back then. I was born into a system that neglected my safety altogether: for being a queer man, for being a political activist and journalist, and for simply being born in Syria, a country that criminalizes homosexuality, in a time of war where humans aren't valued at all. In a country where people are dying by the thousands, a gay person is easy prey, and unlikely to see justice.

I survived in Lebanon as a Syrian refugee for two years the same way I survived the Arab world for the twenty-eight years before that: I built walls around me. They got higher with every challenge I faced: I was fired from a job I loved for being gay, I was gay-bashed by people I thought were my friends. Those walls protected my identity, protected who I am, and held my sexuality—alongside my aspirations, my dreams and hopes for the future—deep within me. This is how I felt safe.

My physical safety was violated so many times that it didn't matter much to me anymore. I never lived in a country where I felt completely and utterly safe. I never slept in a house where I didn't jump out of bed at the calmest of whispers. I never walked in a dark street where I didn't stare at people's eyes, fearing that they might be able to see through mine, to tell that I'm queer.

Being an LGBTQ person in the Arab world is not a challenge you face every now and again. You face it every day, feeling unsafe in almost every context. Like children lost in the woods, every sound is a bear attacking, every pair of fireflies is the haunting eyes of a crouching wolf.

Building those walls around me back in the Middle East was the only coping mechanism possible. I couldn't control the world around me, I couldn't change the whole society, I didn't have a single place that I considered safe. I had three possible options: freeze, fight, or flight. After many frozen moments of fear and endless fights that I never won, I decided to fly. I packed my bags, carried my walls in my soul, and I made it all the way to Canada ... to safety.

For the first couple of months after I arrived, I somehow forgot about those walls, or maybe they forgot about me. I unpacked my bags and excitedly explored Vancouver. Life was bright, happy, calm, and tickling to the point of giggles. I slept with both of my eyes closed, and drifted into the land of dreams uninterrupted. Mornings came with the smell of Turkish coffee. They felt sweet, like a funny pet sleeping in your bed and licking your face to wake you up every morning.

This might seem like a happy ending for a Syrian queer refugee story, but it's not.

It turned out I didn't leave my walls behind; they came here with me. Vancouver's lingering winter brought with it a lack of sun, the desperate search for a job, and a newcomer's loneliness. My walls were on alert; they knew they should protect me.

They just didn't know how.

The smell of coffee in the morning began to make me anxious, the short conversations I had with strangers felt pushed and inauthentic, the beautiful city I moved to felt dark and taunting and trapping. I had a difficult time integrating into the Canadian LGBTQ community; it felt like everyone else knew the steps to the Canadian social dance, simply syncing to each other's conversations while I danced on my own. When I immigrated, I left behind the staring eyes, taunting whispers, and dangerous streets, but I also left behind every meaningful relationship I had, every source of solace I built for myself. My sense of belonging to a community was threatened; my self-determination was shattered to pieces. I completely lost trust in myself. The walls I'd built to protect myself from homophobia and to stop others from hurting me felt heavier and denser. Safety never came.

My counsellor didn't pick up on any of that. Bless her; she tried. She tried to calm me down, she tried to help me overcome those anxious moments, and to find peace. But she didn't understand that those fears were rooted within me, that those walls weren't built upon arriving here in Canada; they were with me all along, hidden in my soul, and simply modified in the face of new challenges. When confronted with danger so foreign to me, the only way I could protect myself was to isolate within my own walls. The more I talked to my counsellor, the more locked-in I felt. So I abandoned counselling, and decided to rely on myself in seeking the mental and physical healing I needed.

Months later, I was still struggling with my mental health. My self-esteem suffered, I struggled with physical pains that I couldn't explain, and I lost lots of weight. My family doctor, himself an immigrant from South Africa, dismissed it all. "You're fine," he told me, pointedly looking at his watch. "It's all normal. Just be normal."

As I walked out of the clinic, I felt dismissed, uncared for, lonely.

Later that fall I found myself at a table full of friends and strangers sharing a Canadian Thanksgiving dinner I'd been talked into attending. I ended up sitting beside a white queer man who worked as a naturopathic doctor. Over the course of the meal, I told him my story. At the end of the night he handed me his card, said he might be able to help.

I'd never been to a naturopath before. The concept seemed funny, like a pseudoscience, but I pushed myself, and decided to try. My first impression was how warm and accessible he was. We talked about comics and superheroes, a queer party we both wanted to go to on the weekend, and our favourite smells. He made me feel comfortable and didn't shy away from exposing his own feelings. He asked me personal questions in a respectful way, understanding my reluctance to answer some of them, and provided alternative ways to express myself.

"How is your libido?" he asked, smiling.

"I've never talked to a doctor about my sexual habits before," I told him, trying to avoid the topic.

"It's all right, that's completely understandable. I would find it weird to speak about my sexual habits to a total stranger," he said. "We can use metaphors if you prefer, or maybe words in your own language that you're comfortable using."

"I'm willing to learn if you're willing to teach me."

We laughed, and I told him about my libido.

Unlike some people I've met who suffered from what I thought of as the White Man Saviour Complex—thinking they knew better than me how to handle my own life and challenged every choice I made—my naturopathic doctor respected my agency.

"These are my recommendations," he said, after a ninety-minute discussion about my mental and physical health. "You're under a lot of stress, which is understandable and expected. I recommend you take these supplements and try them for a month."

He told me to report back to him every week via text and tell him how I felt. "We will work together on adjusting them according to you," he said warmly. "We will decide together on the best road to take."

His office felt like a safe space where I was respected for who I was. He saw me as a unique individual with agency and self-determination, and that felt good.

Taking care of my health with the help of a naturopath felt like the first step on the right path, but I knew that stress had left physical as well as mental scars on me. It felt like someone was strangling me from behind, hands wrapped around my throat all the time, forcing me still. My naturopath helped care for my inner body, but he couldn't cure this physical pain. I realized that I needed more help.

I'd never been to a massage therapist before, and I had to convince myself to go. *It's for rich and powerful men, and I'm not sure how I will feel when a stranger touches me that way.* But I soon found one who made me feel at ease. He was a person of colour from Hawaii, funny and encouraging. Like me, he knew how uncomfortable it feels to be treated as "exotic" and reduced to a stereotype. He respected me and supported me from that perspective. He told me about his own life and his own culture, and was interested in knowing more about my own.

We never talked about the war in Syria. He's the only person who didn't persist in asking me to detail my experiences as a refugee. Instead, he treated me like any other person, and that was exactly what I needed. He worked my tense muscles, untying knots in my system that I didn't even realize were there. Under the pressure of his fingers, I felt the muscles. They were tense, short, and strangling. With practiced touch, he followed the muscle fibers up and down my neck, while explaining to me the many stretches that would help reduce the tension there.

I wanted to know what was happening to my body, and he was generous with his knowledge. I felt safe, content, and trusting.

Between my naturopath and my massage therapist, I began to feel the positive benefits that these two health professionals had on my entire life. My comfort level started to grow within me, big enough for me to go back to counselling. My anxieties used to feel like a random herd of sheep rampaging around my brain. But with the support of my holistic Dream Team, I was able to corner those sheep, and felt ready to examine them with a counsellor again.

In the first session with my new counsellor, an Indigenous woman who specialized in trauma and grief, I told her about my past experience with counselling. She listened to me intently, then asked me to listen to her. "You're a smart person, and you're good at self-reflection," she told me. "You need a counsellor who realizes that, and who is able to outsmart you."

It was true: I was very protective of myself. She saw the walls I'd built around me for years, and she was willing to climb them, and to challenge me in the process.

It's not about breathing techniques. It's not about easy answers. It's about digging deep and finding the person I am. Every session with her feels painful, as if she is peeling burned skin off my body. My counsellor speaks a language I understand: logic. She sees the real reasons why I feel the way I do and she aims to discover the causes of my discomfort. She chips at the foundations on which my walls are built.

And it's working. Her work feels like the wind hitting a mountain: it might not move it today, but it sure as hell will break it one grain of sand at a time.

I used to feel like the world was falling down on me, like a child trapped under the rubble of my reality and surviving on the tiny bits of air I could grasp. Now, I hear my Dream Rescue Team telling me to hold on, and I know I'm on my way to finally feeling safe.

QUEER AND TRANS HEALTH INNOVATION PROFILE

Access Alliance Multicultural Health and
Community Services LGBTQ+
Newcomer Initiatives (Toronto, Ontario)

Ranjith Kulatilake, Community Health Worker

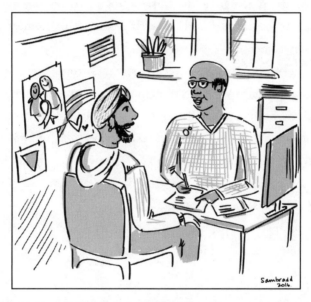

*Tell us about Access Alliance's LGBTQ+ Newcomer Initiatives and
why you're proud of them.*

Access Alliance is a community health centre that provides primary health care, community health programs, and interpreter services for immigrants and refugees in Toronto, with specialized services for LGBTQ+ newcomers that include resettlement support workshops, one-on-one sessions, and prioritized access to primary health care. We're some people's first point of contact when they arrive in Canada. We help them become reintegrated, find employment, and become very settled here.

One of our core programs is a series of weekly resettlement workshops specifically for LGBTQ+ newcomers. The workshops provide a safe and inclusive space for LGBTQ+ newcomers of varied status: refugee claimants, refugees, permanent residents, and Canadian citizens. They cover many topics related to LGBTQ+ resources, mental, physical, and sexual health, Canadian culture, housing, and employment. Newcomer volunteers lead in organizing the space, sometimes presenting or co-presenting. Here they can safely share expertise, build leadership skills, and connect with other LGBTQ+ newcomers.

These workshops are held weekly at our Toronto East location, and monthly at our Toronto West location. In the past three years more than 125 workshops have been conducted with over 2,000 attending, cumulatively.

One-on-one sessions for resettlement services are also available at these locations. More than 200 of our LGBTQ+ newcomer clients have gained convention refugee status over the past three years and are given priority access to the agency's clinical services.

Every summer we celebrate Pride at our East and West locations with LGBTQ+ newcomers leading in organizing, presenting, and celebrating their journeys.

What changes are you trying to create? What problems are you trying to solve? What does success look like?
Services for LGBTQ+ newcomers are uncommon in the health sector. There are fewer than ten similar programs in all of Ontario. Transphobia, homophobia, racism, social isolation, intricate system navigation, and culture shock, for example, are unique social determinants of health for them, and are taken into account in our interdisciplinary and anti-oppressive approach.

High levels of client satisfaction, increasing numbers of LGBTQ+ newcomers accessing our services, and successes in their resettlement and reintegration define the success of our programs.

If someone from another place emailed you to say, "I want to do this in my community," and asked for your advice on how to do it, what would you tell them?

Service providers often say, "We don't have LGBTQ+ clients." Even by conventional standards, 10 percent of the general population is queer. If they have not come out, it is primarily because the service providers have not reached out to them and not facilitated safer, welcoming, comfortable environments. Thus it is necessary to include queer positivity in every program, in every space that you want to serve the public.

In order to sustain such an approach, a policy must be established that recognizes the social determinants of health for LGBTQ+ newcomers, to advocate within and outside the agencies to eradicate barriers that exist, and to train staff regularly. Rainbow flags and posters should be displayed within spaces to make these newcomers feel welcome, otherwise a space can be heteronormative and sometimes heterosexist. At Access Alliance, English and French posters proclaim, "You are a part of our community. This is an LGBTQ+ and newcomer positive space." We also have all-gender washrooms.

If your organization was gifted $1 million (with no strings attached) by a donor, and your success was completely guaranteed, what would you choose to do?

I would create a resource centre for LGBTQ+ newcomers where they could just be themselves, learn more about LGBTQ+ people, and access employment and resettlement resources. I would also create an emergency fund to help people pay for food or transport, or to send money home if a loved one is in need. Many LGBTQ+ newcomers were the breadwinners in their home countries, and their lives don't stop when they come to Canada.

For more information about Access Alliance's LGBTQ+ Newcomer Initiatives, visit accessalliance.ca

No blood test can detect grief or disgrace. No research survey can quantify the harmful impact of having your queer communities—your so-called safe, inclusive spaces—other you again and again.

SEX WORK SOLIDARITY AS HEALING

in four parts

Amber Dawn

1. Trust Exercise

One upon a time ... in fact, I'm referencing 1996, but maybe the familiarity of a faerie tale intro will thwart the standard dubiety or "othering" that occurs when a sex worker speaks up. Othering is the means through which sex workers are rendered into makeshift statistics within countless shelved reports. Othering is how sex workers' voices are dismissed as the most current legislation governing prostitution is being passed (C-36 in Canada, for example). Moreover, othering is an everyday mindset that pervasively allows negative perceptions of sex workers to be openly asserted, as in: we are heteronormative family wreckers, criminals, disease spreaders, drains on the system, victims, patriarchy perpetuators; even some cisgendered and trans queer circles see us as inconvenient obstacles to mainstream acceptance.

Before reading this essay about accessing appropriate health and wellness care as a sex worker, I'm going to ask you to reflect on your own relationship to othering—perpetuating, witnessing, and surviving it—and how it has impacted your health. You're reading *The Remedy*, and if I take this as a clue, I can imagine that aspects of your own identity have been ousted by the dominant mainstream, and maybe othering has literally sickened you.

Solidarity work is much more complicated than "we're all in this fight together" kind of thinking, of course. I'd like to share some personal and practical knowledge that I've learned about how to solidarize with sex workers. And sex workers need close allies. Not "for the sake of the argument" close or "save the less fortunate" close, but "eye-to-eye" close. To encourage this closeness, I will invite you to participate in self-reflection, seek-and-find games, holistic intervention, and yes, I'll use faerie tale phrasing ... *Once upon a time*, in 1996, a family physician was seeing a patient for the first time. This patient disclosed that she was violently raped by a bad date while working on the street and since then she's had difficulty managing back and leg pain, sleeping, eating, and concentrating. This patient said, "I've only had shitty experiences with doctors. What can you tell me that will help me trust you?"

Now imagine you are that family physician or that nurse, that social worker, that clinical supervisor, health care researcher, emergency room receptionist, front line shelter worker, LGBTQIA hotline volunteer, that confidant or lover or friend. What would you say to help build trust?

And indeed trust has been broken. I am not the only sex worker who has waited anxiously in a doctor's office while brooding over scores of "shitty" previous experiences. A 2014 survey—the *Street Based Sex Worker Needs Assessment*—led by a research team of former sex workers in Toronto, Barrie, and Oshawa, Ontario, showed that a quarter of the interviewees almost never see a health care provider, while nearly half rarely or never disclose their involvement in sex work to their health care provider. Judgmental health care and social service providers were the most prominent concern mentioned by interviewees.

This is painfully similar to a 2005 survey—*Social Determinants of Health Care Access Among Sex Industry Workers in Canada*—conducted in cities in British Columbia where many sex workers reported feeling intimidated and shamed by health care professionals, and chose to withhold information relevant to their health care due to fear of discrimination. Similar again to a discussion paper—*Addressing Sex Workers' Risk for HIV/AIDS*—presented at the 1996 International Conference on AIDS, which examined how sex workers have historically been disinclined to access health and social services on account of the stigma associated with their occupation.

I've gathered countless testimonials myself, not as a researcher, but as a co-worker and friend. There was the parlour worker who teared up in the staff room as she recounted a recent STI test where the nurse startled her by attempting to insert a swab up her anus before she had finished taking down her pants. The escort whose examination was interrupted by a half dozen medical students, none of whom greeted her, used her name, or acknowledged that she could hear them while they discussed her profession and diagnosis. The street worker who warned me about a particular receptionist at the free clinic—a receptionist that had said, "You people are always sick," and made her wait indefinitely without giving her an appointment number. And there is me; the "shitty" experience I remember most clearly is being told by a hospital psychiatrist that "the human spirit can only take so much" and "if you continue down your path, there will be no recovery."

Once upon a time in 1996, that family physician addressed my question about trust by saying, "I believe you. I'm sorry this happened to you. With your permission, I'd like to run some physical exams ..."

2. (Make) Believe

We are fourteen women gathered around a conference table to train as volunteers at an anti-violence feminist crisis line. Together we are brainstorming how to respond when a caller discloses rape or violence. "I believe you" is written in black marker on flip chart paper. "I believe you" has likely been written on flip charts by anti-violence feminists for decades. "I believe you" is the first step in countervailing victim-blaming and social scrutiny of survivors' stories. It is a non-judgmental precursor to active listening, offering resources and supporting the survivor's choices for healing. I am grateful to the feminists who taught me to believe.

My gratitude is tainted, however, by the number of times I've been forced to defend my commitment to anti-violence work to abolitionist feminists—who intentionally confuse sex work with trafficking and violence against women. Abolitionists who aim to keep (or make) sex work illegal, and further still who propose to see sex work no longer exist in any form. This is both ludicrous—as sex work will always exist—and glaringly paternalistic and condescending towards sex workers' individual and community autonomy.

The abolitionist argument alone is exhausting enough, but the real damage occurs when abolitionist feminists staff support services that sex workers may need. For example, I have witnessed a white feminist front-line worker tell an Asian sex worker that she could stay at the emergency women's shelter *as long as* she recognized that sex work isn't work, it should never be called work, only abuse.

Would you want to access a support service where a fundamental part of your lived experience was discredited at the front door? "I believe you" has a beginning and an end. Too often sex workers are not believed—and we are not believed by the very services and organizations that claim to uphold the phrase "I believe you."

3. Seek-and-Find

I have something in common with the British Columbia workers' compensation board: a fondness for seek-and-find pictures. My favourite page of WorksafeBC.com is "What's wrong with this photo?" where you can seek-and-find hazards in various occupational scenarios. For example, a photo of a landscaping scenario shows one worker wearing flip-flops while pushing a lawn mower, and another appears to be texting while climbing a ladder. This is observational learning.

Sex workers are excellent observational learners; however, I have yet to discover a "What's wrong with this photo?" of a sex workplace scenario. Let's create one now. I'll give you a scenario—a real and personal account—and you try to find the risks and the harm-reduction activities. Ready?

A client waits for me in the massage room. I haven't seen him before although he is a frequent regular at the parlour. As I grab my trick bag of condoms, water-based lube, and alcohol-free disinfecting wipes, a co-worker informs me this client uses cocaine. "Beware of coke dick," are her exact words. In the massage room the client has set up a few lines of coke on the night stand beside the money he's set out for my tip. Normally, I collect my tips quietly, but as the client offers me his coke straw, I roll up a bill and say, "I've always fantasized about snorting coke through a hundred-dollar bill." Minutes later we are naked and covered in massage oil. The client repeatedly squirts oil from the bottle onto my breasts and we both laugh like this is the funniest thing to ever happen. In my mind, I curse the recent trend in "oiled up" porn (fucking oil!). I slide my body over his, being careful, though not as careful as I could be, of any pre-cum leaking from his limp penis. When he gets an erection, he grabbles eagerly for a condom. "Let me do that, baby," I say. I stick my ass in his face, talk dirty to him, and play with his balls as

I hastily wipe some oil off my hands and get a condom on him. He groans and pounds his fists on the wall in frustration as his erection wavers.

How many did you find? You could find up to fifteen depending on how you tally up risk and safety. Condoms and water-based lube are easy to spot. Alcohol-free wipes are included as safer sex supplies because isopropyl alcohol weakens condoms, as does massage oil. There is a low risk of Hep C infection from sharing coke straws. There are lower concentrations of HIV in pre-cum than in semen. Even Dr. Google will give you this information. What may be less seek-and-findable is the immeasurable safety of working together. In this scenario, I am with other workers inside a parlour where we can exchange information about clients. How would the risks increase if I were alone and high with a new client who was growing frustrated?

Sex workers are excellent observational learners not just because our occupation requires us to be hyper attentive to what's happening around us, but also because ultimately we depend on each other to model safer work practices. Criminalization, full or asymmetrical, and other systemic barriers that prevent sex workers from working together and freely sharing information amongst ourselves puts our health at risk. It not only impedes on our ability to learn from each other, it increases the likelihood that police will refuse to protect sex workers, and instead will routinely confiscate condoms from street and massage parlour workers as evidence of criminal activity. Indeed, this is already happening. It means that outreach services, like mobile health vans, will face additional limitations in getting safer sex and harm reduction supplies to sex workers who need them. Criminalization fractures sex workers from each other and from appropriate health services. I will say it here, and likely countless times in the future: if you want to be an ally, support decriminalization.

There are several sex worker-led organizations in Canada that provide information about decriminalization and sex work justice. A few from coast to coast include: PEERS Victoria, PACE Vancouver, Maggie's Toronto, Big Susie's Hamilton, Power Ottawa, Stella Montreal, Stepping Stones Halifax. Friends in the USA and internationally, the Bay Area Sex Worker Advocacy Network (BaySwan) keeps an excellent list of organizations on their website. And from any location, *Tits and Sass*, a group blog run by sex workers, is my absolute favourite online read.

Supporting decriminalization can take many forms. You might host a potluck fundraiser or dance party to raise some donation money for an organization. Invite some friends over for a write-in and compose letters to local senators or government officials, or co-author an op-ed for your local paper or political blog. Why not volunteer (contribute to the cause and also you might meet cute workers or allies)? Share petitions and information on social media. Become so darn articulate that you could readily speak up for sex workers' rights within your own communities. Be an outspoken, bad-ass, sex worker ally at an upcoming dinner party—try it!

4. Holistic Intervention

In a land far, far away … in fact, I'm referencing a recent queer dance party held in a warehouse located along one of Vancouver's last street-working strolls. Like any queer dance party, a good number of the party-goers, myself included, were hanging around outside to air our sweaty bodies or smoke or flirt with sweaty smokers. A gorgeous queen in daisy dukes sauntered over to the curb and pretended to hustle; her friends hooted at her. My chest tightened. This party was located six-and-a-half blocks from where I was violently raped by a bad date.

Some femme shouted, "No, honey, you are way prettier than the hookers around here." My temples began to ring. Three blocks away was where Sheila Catherine Egan was last seen. One block away was where Jennie Furminger was last seen. I remember their names because I remember them. Sheila was two years younger than me. Jennie was born and raised in my hometown. Is this how they shall be spoken of—as "ugly hookers"—by queer kids stopping by the stroll for a cheap place to drink and dance?

"Don't you ever insult the women in this neighbourhood," I said, my voice raised.

Everyone around me froze. The femme eyed her friends pleadingly like she was looking for back-up. "It was just a joke," she said.

I lay into her again, "Don't you ever—"

No blood test can detect grief or disgrace. No research survey can quantify the harmful impact of having your queer communities—your so-called safe, inclusive spaces—other you again and again. To be othered by anti-sex worker comments or "jokes" stings, certainly. What cuts deeper is the othering of having no one stand beside you. No one offered a single word of solidarity in that moment—and that moment is by no means a unique example. At times, this has caused me to see other queers as potential threats to my dignity and well-being, and it has also caused me to isolate from queer communities altogether.

There are always ways to intervene against othering. When I say "intervention" I'm not talking about those pop-sensational reality shows about addiction, I'm talking about holistic and preventative care. The healing properties of allyship also cannot be measured by medical assessment, but they are equally real. And we must believe we can heal from the sickness and damage. Staging an intervention against othering requires some planning. The greatest care an ally may offer is simply to be ready to speak up and stand with sex workers. I offer the following examples:

A friend calls me the day before the International Day to End Violence Against Sex Workers and asks if I'd like her to march in the red umbrella procession with me, and should she call other friends so I have an ally posse.

A professor in the creative writing program where I now work performs a pro-decriminalization themed TEDx Talk called *The red umbrella—sex work, stigma, & the law*, and forwards the YouTube link to all of our colleagues. I sit in my cubicle with awe as I read thoughtful and affirming replies coming in from nearly every professor and staff member. Being "out" at work becomes more secure in a matter of hours.

A friend joins me each year to host a fundraiser cabaret for the Missing and Murdered Women's March. Together we gather a group of queer artists who volunteer their time and talent to raise money for the Aboriginal and community elders and families of the missing and murdered women in Vancouver. Sometimes I keep the donation money in my bra before delivering it to the elders—just for old times' sake.

My wife takes the morning off work to go to a sensitive doctor's visit with me. She says, "I can wait in the lobby or come into the exam room?" and "I can help you vocalize your concerns to the doctor or I can support you quietly?" and "Afterwards, can I take you to that fried chicken place you like?" and she says, "I love you. I'm with you."

And that family physician from *once upon a time* in 1996 happens to be a lesbian doctor. After years in family medicine, she moved into a different field of care, but I still see her from time to time at queer events. She greets me with professional discretion, yet also undeniable warmth. I will forever remember her saying, "I believe you."

And right now, you are reading my words. I thank you for your kind attention and your solidarity. Never forget that you too can do this healing work.

Queers have always used flagging—subtle codes invisible to non-community members but visible within the community—as signifiers of belonging and identity so that we know how to spot each other in a mixed crowd … As queer psychotherapists, we offer our own version of flagging, cueing our clients before they walk into our offices that we are a safe place for them to bring their whole selves, and that we might have some community affiliation and knowledge.

THE DISCLOSURE OF SPECIALIZATION

A QPOC Therapist's Questions about Embodied Mirroring and Mentoring

Keiko Lane

Author's note: In case examples from my clinical practice, clients' identities and details are changed significantly to disguise their specificity and identity. The issues raised are actual questions and issues from my clinical practice, supervision, and teaching.

As I held the door open for Maria and welcomed her into my office for our first appointment, she paused briefly and scanned the bookshelves closest to the door. It isn't uncommon for new clients to stop and look at the books. That's why they are there: Minnie Bruce Pratt, Cherrie Moraga, Audre Lorde, S. Bear Bergman, Essex Hemphill, Patrick Califia, Joy Harjo, Paul Monette, *This Bridge Called My Back*, anthologies of Black queer writing, Asian American feminists, and the first few issues of *Transgender Studies Quarterly*.

It used to be that in large urban areas such as California's Bay Area where I practice, clients came to psychotherapy not knowing anything about the therapist with whom they were entering a relationship other than our name and address, and maybe a few things told to them by the friend or health practitioner who had referred them to us. That was before the internet, websites, and social media.

As Maria sat down on the couch opposite my chair, she looked at me and said, "I wondered if you would look like your pictures."

"And do I?" I asked her, not sure where this was going.

"Yes," she said, smiling a little.

"You look glad about that."

"Yes," she said. "I was looking for a queer femme of colour. But it's complicated, because I'm mixed. White femmes don't see me, but femmes of colour sometimes don't see me either. I know you're mixed. And in your photos you look mixed, like, chameleon-like, sort of? In some photos you look Asian, in others, you look more white. So I figured you would get it. You do get it, right?"

There were so many pieces of information in this brief introduction that I didn't know where to start. I wasn't sure what she needed from me.

"You thought I'd get what it's like to not be recognized fully?" I asked her.

"Yeah," she said, looking suddenly shy and away from me.

"Yeah," I said, "I do." While I waited for her to look up, I took in her features—long dark hair, brown eyes, light skin. She was petite, wearing black jeans and a blue sweater, black sandals, and red lipstick. She finally looked up at me and smiled, then covered her mouth.

"You probably think that was pushy of me to ask. Or intrusive. I don't mean to intrude, I just have been looking for someone who gets it." Suddenly she had tears in her eyes.

She began to tell me her story. She was in her late twenties. Her mother was Mexican-American and her father was Irish-American, and she had moved to the Bay Area a year earlier with her partner, a white transman whom she met when they were in college. They had moved so that he could go to law school, and she was working as an administrator at a large nonprofit.

Maria had come to therapy because she was having trouble connecting with new community. She and her partner John had a large community in the college town where they had met, but upon moving to the Bay Area John had come to a place in his transition where he was seeking to pass as male full time. Maria understood and wanted to support him, but felt that his passing as male, in conjunction with his whiteness, left her invisible when they were out in the world as a couple.

Maria had especially sought out a therapist who she thought would understand her. She thought that I could help her feel less invisible and more connected. Maria's research into my background and her hopeful assumptions based on that information made me think about flagging.

Queers have always used flagging—subtle codes invisible to non-community members but visible within the community—as signifiers of belonging and identity so that we know how to spot each other in a mixed crowd. Some flagging is conscious—hankies, clothing, the queer iconography of ACT UP and Queer Nation stickers in the 1990s, the ways we use social media and websites to explicitly name our cultural locations in the world—and some flagging is unconscious—the inflection in our voice when we talk, the ways our bodies inhabit space, and whose bodies our eyes linger on as we walk down the street.

Part of the work of psychotherapy is to make the unconscious conscious. Part of the work of queer psychotherapy is to make our queer embodied signifiers conscious, to make choices about what we flag, when and how we present, and explore how we feel about it. We look for models, mentors, and mirrors. As queers, we usually don't find our queerness modeled in our parents. We look outside of our families of origin for other queers.

Sometimes we look at our therapists. In psychoanalytic terms, we call this transference. In queer cultural terms, we might call it an unconscious seeking out of models and mentorship.

As queer psychotherapists, we offer our own version of flagging, cueing our clients before they walk into our offices that we are a safe place for them to bring their whole selves, and that we might have some community affiliation and knowledge. Maria had looked me up and on my professional clinical website found my bio that announced my identity in the world as a mixed-race queer, photos in which my long hair and lipstick out me as one version of femme, and links to my professional writing in which I talk about intersections of racial and gender justice.

Especially for LGBTQIA clients who are also POC and/or HIV+ and who often straddle multiple sites of exclusion, the desire for a therapist who mirrors their identities can feel urgent and crucial. And for therapists the desire to be seen can also enter into the relational realm. As clinicians, naming a specialization is naming a deep relationship to a particular identity, experience, or cultural location. Clients often hope that the relationship is sameness. Sometimes it is, and sometimes it is deep alliance and affiliation. The client's hope of twinship and the therapist's hope of service and being seen leave each vulnerable to the other. This can be fertile ground for deep therapeutic work, and it can also lead to assumptions and disappointments.

After Maria left my office at the end of our first session, I wondered how much of her experience of isolation was new and how much of it was familiar. She had sought me out because she wanted someone who would understand her experience. And she was both correct and incorrect. As a mixed-race femme who is often assumed to be white and straight, I do understand the anxieties of invisibility, the ways in which the politics of exclusion trigger fears of not being a good enough QPOC community member by virtue of invisibility projected from other people. But there would certainly be ways in which our experiences didn't overlap. She had told me what her hopes were. I wondered what would happen when I inevitably disappointed her.

Over the next few months, Maria and I worked with her experiences of being seen and unseen in the world and in her intimate relationships. When I asked Maria to talk about times when she felt visible, she was silent.

"I can't think of any," she said, looking sad.

"You can't think of any times when you have felt seen?" I reflected back.

"Well, a little bit. Here and there. But never the whole story all at once. I mean, with John, he sees me. I know he loves me. But it's like when we're out in the world together and he's passing as male, which he is, he forgets that it means I'm passing as straight, which I'm not. So, it isn't that he doesn't know who I am, but it's like we can't both be fully present at the same time. And my family, well, both of my parents like to point out the ways I look like my dad's family. Everyone thinks that I will have an easier time in life if I pass."

"So with your family you pass as white, and with John you pass as straight."

"Yeah."

"What does passing mean?"

She looked at me, a little confused.

I continued. "Well, of course passing is in part about what people see, right? Do they see your light skin, or your lipstick and long hair? But we also embody ways of being that signify affiliations. For example, when you and John met, how did he know that you were queer and not just a straight girl?"

Her eyes lit up. "Oh! I wanted his attention." She laughed. "I knew who he was—the big queer on campus, and I thought he was hot. I was trying to get him to notice me."

I laughed with her. "So what did you do? How did you get his attention?"

"I probably was strutting a little, making sure he'd notice."

"And he did, obviously."

She smiled, her eyes lighting up at the memory.

"So what's different now?"

"I don't know," she said, frowning.

In body-oriented, or somatic, psychotherapy, we think about body-felt reflections. We feel and explore our bodies as we move through the world. We also think of social justice in terms of bodily proximity to power and survival. Which bodies are given what kinds of attention in the world? Which bodies are eroticized? Which bodies are criminalized? Which bodies are assumed to occupy locations of power or privilege? What embodiments and ranges of movement do we understand and process as signifiers of which social locations?

Part of the work in psychotherapy is to bring attention and awareness to the body and then begin to consciously shape our movements through the world. So we set up an experiment and Maria began walking around my office. At first she walked the way she moved through the world on her own. I asked her to notice where she felt energy in her limbs and her core, and where she didn't; where she could feel her breath. Then she moved around the room in the same way as when she was with John, then in the same way she as when she was trying to get his attention when they first knew each other. She moved back and forth between the three embodiments, then stood still and looked at me.

"Oh, it's like my energy is, well, not gone entirely, but subdued."

"What does it feel like?"

"Sort of numb, like I forgot about me."

We were both quiet for a moment, taking in her statement.

"So how would you like to feel, to be aware of yourself taking up space in the world?"

Over the next few sessions, we worked on her sense of her embodied self. She walked around the room as we talked, and tried different postures as she sat on the couch. Then one day she said, "There isn't a mirror in here. I can't see the differences. I can feel them, but I don't know what they look like. Will you do them with me, show me how I'm moving?"

I began moving with her, mirroring her movements. She gave me instructions on how to follow her, and she watched me as we moved around the room together.

After a few minutes of this, we sat back down. She was silent and looking away from me.

"How was that?" I asked her.

"Well, I could see the differences in how I move, and it helped me to feel the different postures and movement." She still wasn't looking at me, which was unusual for her.

"What else?"

"Well," she said, still averting my gaze, "when you were moving the way I directed you, following my movement, you looked so different from the way you usually look. I thought that maybe both could be true, that we would look the same, and that you would also still look the way you always look."

In psychoanalytic terms, we would call this twinship transference: a desire for sameness. In queer cultural terms we recognize Maria's desire echoing from the first session of wanting to feel seen, and now we understand that it isn't just being seen that she craves, it's being the same. She is disappointed that I am not the same as she is. This is the conflict between us that I had anticipated. I had disappointed her in revealing our differences. And her desire and disappointment are familiar to my own experience as a mixed-race femme—a desire to be both seen and mirrored—to not feel alone in my identity.

I want to comfort her. And I want to tell her all of the ways that I think we are similar. But jumping over her sadness and frustration is a political temptation about showing alliances. The psyche is messy and doesn't always match our politics.

Queering psychotherapy means questioning and subverting the traditional boundaries of psychoanalysis. We are not blank slates. Even without our websites and social media, even without Google searches and writing for online journals, we are visible to each other. We recognize that power is always present in the room between us and in the world and we struggle to make sense of it together. We each shape our bodies in relationship to our internalized scripts of bodily possibility. We recognize in each other the shape of possibility.

I tell all of this to Maria. Together we grieve her experience of loneliness. We wonder how it might be part of the inherent experience of mixed-race identity and of queerness, that we must find our own way. That the best we can do and offer to each other is a model of possibility about how one finds one's way, but the actual embodied path is unique. As we talk about it, we think that maybe that is really what being human is, but queerness quickly strips away the illusion of sameness.

In psychotherapy, we talk about the idea of the good enough therapist—that we do our best to provide what our client needs, and in the spaces where we fail, we stay close to our clients and help them develop resilience and tolerance of the inevitable failures of those who care for them. I wonder if queering psychotherapy also means being a good enough mirror—knowing that while we cannot provide our clients with their desired map of queer survival or identity, we can reflect back to them their sorrows, strengths, and resilience as they, and we, find our own way.

... we spend so much time and energy convincing non-trans people of the truth that we are a vulnerable and victimized population to such an extent that sometimes we forget also how fucking strong and resilient we are. These things can exist in tandem: recognition of the injustices against us and also celebration of the fortitude it takes for each of us to live in this world.

TRANS GRIT
Cooper Lee Bombardier

On the mild Sunday evening I became a trans curmudgeon, I sat circled up with two-dozen others in folding chairs: all on a spectrum of gender in the neighbourhood of my own. We ranged in age from high school to near-retirement. Many a year or less into transition, or else trying to decide whether or not to swing a leg over in this rodeo at all. I wasn't seeking support so much as a sense of connection, to be among others like me. Strange to progress from the constant of change to this *olde-trans* status with no segue, no half-time show. All flux, and then it was everything else in life that I needed to deal with.

A young trans guy, anxious and lost in a mass of too-big clothes, shared with utter despondency that someone from a doctor's office was *rude* to him on the phone. He'd crumbled in the face of rudeness, his forward process stymied by the molasses of agonism, this ticket-taker saying: *you're too short to ride, sorry.* He'd hung up the phone, unable to access the care he needed.

Welcome to the rest of your life as a transsexual, I wanted to say. I slouched in my plastic chair like a delinquent student. A cascade of similar tales ricocheted around the room from other younger folks, volleyed in a manner that precluded any true listening or reflection.

You think rudeness *is the worst of it?* I thought, *Microaggressions? You cannot wither in the face of those who don't want to help you. You'll need to learn how to either charm them into being your greatest proponent or else clamp your will to their pant legs with the persistence of a pitbull until they help you!*

Voilà! In an instant I'd become that guy: olde-trans. *A goddamn trans curmudgeon.* Perhaps I no longer belonged at a meeting if I couldn't brim with empathy for the plight of this kid and his vexing phone call. Perhaps the agony, excitement, and wanting a high-five for each achievement, for me, was long gone. I joined this rodeo a decade and a half ago, and my ass was sore from years of rough riding. I was well aware of the judgment that stewed in me and how little my Buddhist practice made a dip in that mucky soup. I wanted to say, across the room, *Buck up, little camper. You're gonna have to be tougher than this. You're gonna need some grit to do this.*

The folding plastic chair chewed at my back as I remembered the hurdles and trials and obstacles and violence and discrimination that trans people I know have overcome for years to be who they are. We were busy confronting and surviving *macroaggressions* and lack of access. I thought of my early mentors who smuggled, shared, and used black-market hormones, or friends who, long ago, lay alone in hotel rooms for a week post-surgery without anyone to help them. People I've met who sought hormones and surgery from doctors twenty, thirty years ago, knapping a wheel out of stone. No Harry Benjamin to jump through, no WPATH to walk. People who turned tricks, went on fertility drugs and sold their eggs, or took out student loans to afford surgery; others who shot street steroids or self-castrated in prison. I thought about trans women friends from the Navajo Nation, who told me stories about pumping parties on the rez where women self-injected hardware-store silicone into their breasts. I thought about a friend whose almost *transmythological* tale about being forced to self-aspirate a hematoma in his chest after top surgery I'd heard about years before we'd ever met, and this was in pre-social networking days. I thought of the countless hours I've spent being told no, that something was unavailable, illegal, or impossible. Or just not right: like a bearded man needing a pelvic ultrasound or mammogram. I thought of the time when, after many years of being on T and procuring top surgery without health insurance, I finally got coverage and then made many long calls appealing to a middle-aged white Texan man at the insurance company to explain why the hysterectomy I was seeking pre-approval for was not part of a not-covered "sex change."

"Look, Hal," I'd explained to this stranger, "I'm not trying to get away with anything here. These are just the parts I was born with, and they're causing me significant pain."

I was frustrated by these young trans people for being so easily discouraged and deterred. If transitioning taught me anything, it was that I needed to possess the will to do whatever it takes to survive.

He held a syringe loose in his hand and with a flick of his hairy wrist threw the point to its hilt into the shiny pocked skin of an orange. *Now you try— hold it like a dart.* He pulled the needle free from the fruit and handed me both. The nervousness in my fingers meant to crush the syringe, but I couldn't crush and dart at the same time. *Exhale.* It took no effort to pierce the rind. I plunged a barrel full of air into the orange. Practice was over. Back in the late '80s, he and his best friend carted black market hormones up from Mexico because there was no clinic back then for guys like us—a practice he has long since disavowed. He, who fucked with the lines in between as creative praxis and sex-art, was my trans lineage, my elder who hewed a clearing for people like me. I lay face down on the bed with my belt and dirty jeans snugged down to the peak of my ass. He directed my girlfriend to push the dart into the meat at the center of a Bermuda triangle found with my hands. My first shot of T, and I chickened out of giving it to myself. The warm oil was a small punch under my skin that might bruise later. *You can do what you want, but I suggest going full-dose at first so you know what it feels like*, he said. And that was the entire point of this whole experiment: for me to know what it felt like to be on Vitamin T. For so long wondering and trying to convince myself I didn't need to. Never being able to really let it go. The anxiety and discomfort and disconnect growing deeper and wider, a canyon cut through the years of a sandstone life, not ever quite fully alive. Now, I would have empirical evidence, a way to compare and contrast. A way to make an informed decision. Once and for all, I hoped. My friend taught me, because thirteen years ago, that's what we had. Just each other.

The modern history of us is so short that we must consciously choose to forget, to unknow, or to never learn in the first place. We are rankled and dogged by the obstacles of systems, protocols, bureaucracies. We peevishly acquiesce to the binary simplicity of the State because it is easier to leave more than breadcrumbs along our paper trails, or else we don't or can't and any minor errand becomes a hassle in having to prove you are real. *I exist, I am possible*, we say, standing right in front of their incredulous/ condescending/confused/irritated faces. A piece of embossed paper seems more real than me in front of you. Standards of care can be problematic, a short leash pulling against our necks. Held up against history, old negatives to the yellow light of a window: before then we got imprisoned, lobotomized, electroshocked, institutionalized. Before and before and before, we existed and we guarded the secret of our existences until our deaths, before that we were burned or drowned, and maybe long before all of that we were revered. Let's always believe that, hold on to that. That maybe once we were respected, like astronauts or creatures that climbed from the froth of the sea to live on land, held in wonder because of the worlds we've straddled and for all of the wisdom we've gathered there in both and in between places.

I worked up the nerve after so many years to cruise into the Tom Waddell clinic in San Francisco's Tenderloin for what we then, with great affection, referred to as Tranny Tuesdays. The trans clinic had opened in the early '90s originally to serve a swath of trans women and trans-feminine people who were being pummeled by AIDS. It was a place that practiced a harm reduction ethos, and prioritized trans people who were sex workers, IV drug users, or surviving on the streets. Even in 2002, it was the only place I knew to go. I waited in a dim hallway in a bucket chair and told the narrative I believed that I had to in order to convince anyone I was trans enough to be on hormones. I would have liked to say that I wanted to know what it was like to be on T so that I could make an informed decision based on experience. It was my first day of many years of saying whatever I had to in the doctor's office to get what I need, and saving my activism for a more systemic approach outside of the examination room. I couldn't fight both battles in the same exact moment.

My doctor tried to reassure me: the lower exam was important, she'd be swift. I told her not to worry because I'd just leave my body anyway. She didn't find this funny, but humour was as vital a survival tool as dissociation was.

I sank against the examination table in my flimsy gown. She came back into the room with Raquel, the physician's assistant, a desert-weathered-handsome middle-aged Hispanic woman from a small Mormon town in Colorado where half the populace was her family. Her people had lived there for two centuries. Raquel flirted while cinching the boa constrictor of the blood pressure cuff around my tattooed bicep. She knew how to strum that chord of making a person feel good and appreciated without hitting the note of implied expectation, the light of a match struck but no fire set. We were from different worlds but found commonalities, like growing up with neighbours who happen to be multiple generations of your family.

I'd never known if Raquel knew I was trans; now, with my bare feet in the cold stirrups and my knees apart, there wasn't much she wouldn't know. My guts gurgled like a clogged toilet, my cheeks flamed with shame. I stared myself away at the composite ceiling tiles until the cold jelly fingers and pain was over. It lasted but two minutes, but time pulled long and thin. After, Raquel came back in with some paperwork. I'd assumed, with no context for someone like me, that her behaviour would change. But she still flirted in her warm way—that day, and as long as she worked there. A year later she will assist my doctor in aspirating a hematoma blooming a purple aquifer in my freshly-sutured-flat chest. The universe knocked me over the head with the cosmic skillet of this lesson: People are so much more willing to understand us than we ever give them credit for. And, that we spend so much time and energy convincing non-trans people of the truth that we are a vulnerable and victimized population to such an extent that sometimes we forget also how fucking strong and resilient we are. These things can exist in tandem: recognition of the injustices against us and also celebration of the fortitude it takes for each of us to live in this world.

I made an appointment with the county clinic for a round of regular STI testing. *Oh, Portland, you trans-nirvana*, I thought, checking off the intake form peppered with a multiverse of sex, gender, sexual orientation, et cetera, et cetera. *Check, check, check!* A clinician went through my intake, asking why I was there and about my various sexual practices. With the tip of her pen she poked a stamp-sized line drawing of a cock and balls at the bottom of the form. "Anything unusual going on for you here? Swelling, itching, sores ... ?"

"Just so you know, I am trans." A silent *Oh!* widened the aperture of her mouth.

"So ... what you're saying is ... this picture doesn't really apply to you."

"Exactly," I say.

She taps my upper arm, trying to recover the blunder. "Well, *good job!* I never would have guessed."

"Well, I *did* check all of the boxes," I say, trying to figure out a non-violent way of informing her that by anointing me with "good job," it implies that there are trans people who are not doing a good job, and that this is highly problematic, because being trans isn't a fucking contest. The clinician is kind, dedicated to community health, and I know she is *doing*, is *trying*, her best. This is what the best looks like in trans-nirvana and I am okay with it because at least I don't feel thwarted, judged, or scared. Patience and willingness to be honest, uncomfortable, to make and transcend mistakes is an arrow that extends in two directions.

The next time I go to the county health office for routine STI testing, I am elated and relieved to discover that my clinician is a trans woman. It's my first time in a medical office where I feel like I can speak all of my truth. I don't need to shuffle my history and pick out the cards I feel I need to show in order to get the treatment I need. I can fan out the whole deck. I don't have to be on guard, or carry it all.

My ass was half-asleep. I hadn't been listening at all to the meeting. It was easier to be frustrated than to look within, because at the bottom of my curmudgeonly feelings was this: *Worry for the very survival of any trans person.* In these memories, just a fraction of many, I held the aggregate of these frictions, this compiled weight. It *is* exhausting. I think this kid, whom I was so quick to judge, maybe had it right all along: We *should* feel annoyed and outraged when we aren't met with helpful service in a medical system we pay so much for in time, energy, and money. And in lives. His distress and frustration at this poor treatment is a probably a good thing; it means we as a demographic have evolved enough to believe *we deserve better*. A momentum started decades before I transitioned is still in a hard swing, the force of which means that now trans people expect a fuck of a lot better. Some things have improved, and still have so much further to go. This road was easier for me because of the suffering, struggle, activism, and work of those who came before me. This kid might one day, thirteen years from now, scoff and roll his eyes hearing about how easy a kid who transitions has it; maybe in 2028 we won't even call it transitioning any more. My trans curmudgeon status might be here to stay, but I realize the kid's expectation for kind helpfulness is a result of trans suffering in the halls of institutionalized medicine, and that his outrage can, and will, become part of a collective lever that ratchets our broken system to a new and better place.

QUEER AND TRANS HEALTH INNOVATION PROFILE

The Trans Buddy Program
(Nashville, Tennessee)

Kale Edmiston, PhD, Co-Founder, and
Lauren Mitchell, PhD, Co-Director

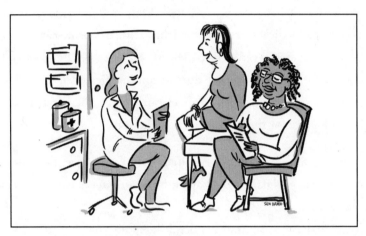

Tell us about the Trans Buddy Program and why you're proud of it.

The Trans Buddy Program pairs trained peer advocates with transgender people seeking health care at Vanderbilt University Medical Center (VUMC) in Nashville. Our volunteers are a diverse and committed group of cis- and transgender people who provide emotional and logistical support to transgender people accessing health care, while facilitating communication between patients and providers.

Because VUMC is a regional leader in health care, we often serve people from across the southeast. Our clients have included adolescents navigating the coming-out process and elder transwomen from rural Tennessee.

What changes are you trying to create? What problems are you trying to solve? What does success look like?

The Trans Buddy Program is improving the health of transgender people by providing a supportive advocate to patients who might otherwise avoid health care. Because many transgender people avoid care due to fears of discrimination and heightened anxiety about medical encounters, Trans Buddy helps reassure patients by putting them in touch with experienced providers, helping them navigate the health care system, and empowering them to become their own self advocates. Our program addresses a lack in an overextended medical system by modeling compassionate care for patients who are often underserved. We alleviate pressure on both sides of the medical visit: for patients, and for doctors and medical staff. For us, success means that an individual patient utilizes our service, then feels empowered enough to advocate for their own health without us.

If someone from another place emailed you to say, "I want to do this in my community," and asked for your advice on how to do it, what would you tell them?

Make sure to have local transgender leadership that has ties to diverse communities on the ground. If program leadership is not connected to the local transgender community, the program will not be utilized by the people who could benefit from it. It is also critical to have relationships with local providers and the support of a health care institution, such as a clinic or hospital.

If the Trans Buddy Program was gifted $1 million (with no strings attached) by a donor, and your success was completely guaranteed, what would you choose to do?

We would start by compensating our wonderful, dedicated volunteers. Then we would hire a diverse trans-identified staff of administrators, clinicians, and social workers to support our missions of outreach, patient care, research, and education. This would include mandatory transgender cultural humility and medical competency training for all providers and staff at our institution, made widely available online, as well as increased outreach to poor, rural, and people-of-colour communities in the Greater Nashville area. We would start a once-a-week "Trans Night" clinic for primary/preventive care in a supportive environment and implement a research project to determine health outcomes for transgender people who utilize Trans Buddy, with an emphasis on adherence, self-efficacy and mental health, and quality of life. Last but not least, a small stipend would be set aside for glitter and rhinestones to fund the decoration of Trans Buddy volunteer vests.

Is there anything else you'd like to tell us?

Direct care work is a different form of social justice activism, where our job is to focus on one-on-one interactions, and to build bridges between individuals and larger institutions. At the core of our work, we assert change through compassion for our clients and their medical providers by offering a stable, patient, knowledgeable presence. We bear witness to stories. We get to remind people that they are deserving of love, care, and support if they forget. It is powerful work.

**For more information about the Trans Buddy Program, visit
medschool.vanderbilt.edu/lgbti/trans-buddy-program**

With only a grim future in my hometown, I knew I would have to leave to become
a whole person. But dislocation would also mean leaving behind the good things,
the security of familiar faces, the abiding beauty of the place. And the river.

RIVERS OF OUR LIVES

Stigma and Dislocations as Part of Life Course

Craig Barron

When I was twelve I lived on the outskirts of a small town in Southern Ontario. There was a beautiful pasture out back and there are photos of me surrounded by horses, looking completely at ease. Further back was a ravine with a spring-fed stream; from there, through some woods, across two fields and an apple orchard, I could be at the door of my public school. On the way I might pass by an enormous pine tree that a friend and I would sometimes climb, wordlessly touching each other's bodies.

The Otonabee River ran through our town and led to a network of shining lakes. My new high school, a just-built brick bunker on twenty-nine acres, overlooked the river. There was a great view through the cafeteria picture windows where I usually sat alone with my fine lunch, always fruit and something fresh-baked brought from home. A good home that I no longer wanted to return to at the end of the day.

I'd stay until closing time in the school library, a two-level room thoughtfully designed with no distracting windows. I found a thick novel about Michelangelo to read, *The Agony and the Ecstasy* by Irving Stone—likely the only available book with content somehow connected to homosexuality.

In grade 10 English class, we read *Huckleberry Finn*. I've kept the essay we were assigned, the question posed: "To what extent is Huck's escape not a rejection of society but a quest for the ideal society?" My profound adolescent words: "Huck was born a type of cast-out from society as the river is so often foreign to the land." Hooked on reading, my imagination would eventually travel from Huck Finn to John Rechy's *City of Night* and Jean Genet—a few interesting detours along the way: *Myra Breckinridge* and *Valley of the Dolls*—places where anything was possible.

Turning sixteen in 1969, I mostly remember being obsessed with a certain boy. I took no notice of historic events like Stonewall, or just months before, the decriminalization of homosexual acts in Canada's criminal code. What I knew was that the risks of articulating love for another boy would have been grave: fear, hatred, rejection, violence; and the stealthy byproducts, the oppressed feelings and crushed identities that are internalized—words like stigma and homophobia not yet part of my vocabulary.

To all appearances our small Kawartha Lakes town was a healthy and secure place for youth. But not gay youth; we simply did not exist. With only a grim future in my hometown, I knew I would have to leave to become a whole person. But dislocation would also mean leaving behind the good things, the security of familiar faces, the abiding beauty of the place. And the river.

The 1970s brought change, the nascent voice of gay liberation, that same-sex love was healthy and natural. But not at home in small towns. Like thousands of others, I saw the mystery and potential of big cities where gay gathering places could be found. With small tentative steps and episodic confrontations, we began to create community in our new homes. In Toronto I was able to visit Glad Day Bookshop's first location in the hallway of a tall dark house in Cabbagetown. Buying a copy of *The Body Politic* became a ritual. Weekend visits to the Manatee Disco.

As a young man alone in a big city, I envisaged real possibilities for a charmed life. But big cities had risks too. I saw damaging temptations, a culture of alcohol and drugs. I met other young gay men with abandoned career ambitions, low self-esteem. Close to the YMCA, I watched Toronto's boys on the streets—prostitution as a rite of passage. I also saw new possibilities for hatred and violence. Jeering Halloween crowds gathered to throw eggs at the gay men in drag leaving the St. Charles Tavern. Though society was making some positive steps—in 1973 the American Psychiatric Association removed homosexuality from its psychiatric disorders list—we were still a massively stigmatized community.

In 1976 my second-storey windows on King Street West overlooked Farb's Car Wash and not much else. Under $200 a month for a two-bedroom apartment. The surrounding buildings were vacant. I remember hanging out a third-floor window with a free-spirited companion and our glasses of wine, an errant group of suburbanites passing by below looking up with disgust. I went to the biggest gay community event of the summer, a dance on the second floor of the Church Street Community Centre: perhaps a hundred people, some awkward dancing to the presumably straight Elton John, and a folksy table laden with plates of carrot sticks and Ritz crackers. The boyfriend that I had dumped months before showed up and informed me that he had bought a house in the Beaches for $40,000—I thought he paid too much. All in all, Toronto depressed me. Time to find another big city.

A place I loved. In 1977 I had acquired a two-room apartment in Montreal's McGill ghetto: French doors and a balcony, a charming old relic of a gas stove in the kitchen, walls that I painted blue. Walking distance to the downtown bars, Le Jardin, the Peel Pub, Le Mystique. An ambiance of tolerance. Culture activities galore. And all those beautiful Montreal men.

I was unprepared for the October early morning phone call from a casual bedmate. He was in prison, one of 145 arrested in the infamous Trux raid. Police had stormed the gay bar armed with machine guns. By nighttime there were 2,000 demonstrators on Ste. Catherine Street. Things quickly unfolded from there; two months later, Quebec became the first Canadian province and one of the first jurisdictions in the world to give human rights protection to gays.

Yes, I was in a good place—but living in a ghetto just the same, the difference between tolerance and acceptance, not part of mainstream society. Building a career and a financial footing, that would be for another day. Five years passed.

One evening in 1982 I was playing Monopoly *en français* with three other gay men. One was particularly aggressive. He wanted it all and he got it all: Rue de la Paix, L'avenue des champs-élysées. But he coughed frequently, had been strangely sick for weeks. Nobody was able to figure it out—or if they had, dared to admit that the mysterious "gay cancer from San Francisco" had arrived.

How quickly the stage was set. In the 1980s AIDS set upon my generation and those younger. And evident from the very start: the stigma when gay sex and death go together, the denial and blame. Turn on the TV in the 1980s and you would get the close-lipped (but still smiling) President Reagan, the bizarre antics of televangelists like Jerry Falwell. An era redolent of war metaphors: AIDS victims who battled with MAI, Toxoplasmosis, Kaposi Sarcoma. And then the warrior drugs like AZT. A *Globe and Mail* columnist wrote that AIDS was taking the most beautiful, the most creative of a generation.

Beside our bookshelf copies of *The Joy of Gay Sex*, we added Paul

Monette's *Borrowed Time* and Larry Kramer's *The Normal Heart*. Then another book, *And the Band Played On*, by Randy Shilts. On staff at Montreal's 1989 V International AIDS Conference, I had a front row view of the media brouhaha surrounding Shilts' story of the hour: Patient Zero, the theory that a gay flight attendant, Gaetan Dugas, had spread AIDS to North America. A complex epidemic reduced to a simple mystery plot: a select collection of data leading to one "promiscuous" gay man. The media loved it; the story now had a villain—everything to do with gay blame and stigmatization and nothing to do with good science.

Gay men and women rallied back, and by the early 1990s AIDS service organizations had become institutionalized. I made my way to Vancouver seeking a healthier environment, trees and ocean breezes. I found work in the education department at AIDS Vancouver. Co-occupants of a downtown building with the BC Persons With AIDS Society (BCPWA, now known as Positive Living), our second-floor offices had their own entrances but shared a photocopier room. Close to my desk it became the backdoor entrance where many young men preferred to enter BCPWA—feeling the stigma of belonging to an "AIDS Society"—and I would pretend not to notice. In HIV prevention for gay men, validating the community was the challenge, being sex-positive a huge part of it. So much about condoms back then, and graphics of HIV continuums, brief time-lines leading from infection to death.

In 1996 Vancouver was home to the XI International AIDS Conference. As a member of the support staff at a planning meeting in Washington, DC, I saw a blank chart on the wall, a program to fill. The organizers were determined that it be a "good-news" conference. And the good news came, reports of a class of new drugs called protease inhibitors. "Manageable disease" became part of the vocabulary. HIV-positive men who had once been told by their doctors that they had six or twelve months to live would soon begin to hear the words "almost-normal life expectancy."

Today in HIV prevention, we have the nuances of undetectable viral load to consider. Treatment as prevention. But it's not all good. The side effects of medications and mental health issues, such as depression, anxiety, survivor guilt, low self-esteem. Ongoing misguided campaigns to criminalize HIV transmission. Ever-enduring stigma.

I am part of a generation that is now middle-aged and older and has seen it all: the name of my boyfriend who I gave up back in 1976 is written on the AIDS memorial beside Toronto's Church Street Community Centre. But we have also thrived: resilience, knowledge, articulation, honesty, and visibility have allowed us to survive as individuals and as a community.

The windows of my old 1970s Toronto apartment today face the entrance to the Toronto International Film Festival, the hub of the theatre district with condominium towers and outdoor restaurant patios. A lot else would once have been beyond my imagination in those days: gay marriage, million-plus attendees at Pride parades, LGBT cultural festivals, openly gay political leaders, health conferences for gay men.

Our health concerns have broadened beyond HIV. Mental illness and substance use can be higher in gay men since we deal with the effects of homophobia and discrimination. Recognizing that good genes and good luck are not enough for good health but that there are also societal influences that have a significant impact. What we call the Social Determinants of Health.

The Public Health Agency of Canada does not consider sexuality among the determinants of health, although we have data in hand showing that gay men are much more likely than straight to have mood or anxiety disorders and significantly greater histories of suicide. We also know that LGBT youth are at a much greater risk of attempting suicide than their straight counterparts. Gay men are also nearly six times more likely to be diagnosed with an STI. Estimates of HIV in the urban gay male population are one in five but one in 1,000 among straight men. Evidently sexuality does determine our health outcomes.

Which brings us to self-care: today, we have more health information and resources available to us than ever before. With greater health literacy, we should have more power over our own health, and more responsibility to evaluate and use these resources—a responsibility shared with our health care providers. But broader social factors affect how people access health services and social supports: Coming out as a life-long process and our personal strategies for coping with stigma. Encountering health care providers limited by homophobia, being treated differently from others. Will gay men who hide their sexuality be comfortable looking for information about their sexual health? Stigma can influence the literacy of both gay men and their health care providers. Mental health will profoundly influence our other health outcomes.

More life dislocations may lie ahead as we search for healthy and secure places to live. Today cities like Toronto, Montreal, and Vancouver are often touted as the world's best places to live. But not everyone has the good life. There is an urgent need for stigma-free shelters for homeless gay youth, some of whom are still rejected by families or bullied in schools. For LGBT people of all ages, the big cities have become an expensive place to live.

For aging gay men, becoming senior citizens, like all older Canadians, means facing the possibility of isolation, a lack of mobility, a loss of one's partner. End-of-life preparations, all that. Today we hear stories of gay seniors being told, of course you will be welcome in senior residences—so long as you keep quiet about your orientation. Or your HIV status, if that is the case. To once again be invisible? Social isolation is perhaps still our greatest challenge.

The river still looks lovely in that small Southern Ontario town and it still has a powerful appeal. But many things have changed: there is a local Gay/Straight Alliance at the high school; there are drag shows. To say nothing about the possibility of a fine rural gay marriage.

Because kindness makes me cry, I burst into tears. Because she isn't a Canadian doctor, she leans in for a hug and I accept it, with gratitude.

SICK OF IT

One patient's adventures in heteronormativity

Caitlin Crawshaw

A nervous receptionist called me on a Friday afternoon to deliver the news. That weird-looking mole on my arm—the one my new GP biopsied *just in case*—was malignant melanoma. As if there's any other kind.

"Do you have someone with you?" she asked. I glanced at my two-year-old daughter upending boxes of toys onto the living room floor and began to cry.

"I'm alone with my toddler," I said between sobs. "My partner's still at work."

"Oh dear! You should have someone with you. Could your husband come home early, maybe?"

I cringed. Not this again.

Five weeks later, my "husband"—common-law wife of ten years—drives me to the cancer hospital in the dawn's early light, holding my hand above the gear shift. I glance behind us at the empty car seat. We've sent the kid to the grandparents while I recuperate from surgery. "I miss her already," I say.

At the hospital, we pass through slow-moving automatic doors and into a dark lobby, where most of the lights are still off. We find the registration desk where a church lady types my information into an aging computer system, staring with knitted eyebrows at the square monitor inches from her bifocals. I glance at the email forward on the wall beside her: it's a letter from "God" to cancer patients, urging them to have faith. Oh boy.

"Last question. Who is your emergency contact?"

"My partner," I say, spelling out G's name slowly. At the last letter, I tense up, preparing for my first dose of intolerance. But without so much as raising an eyebrow, she hands me a green piece of paper with my itinerary. First stop: radiology.

In a basement room, I change into a hospital gown and surrender my street clothes—and dignity—to G for safekeeping. Then I lay sunny-side up on a metal platform. On one side, G squeezes my hand; on the other, a radiologist holds a cartoonishly large metal syringe containing blue, radioactive dye. "This might sting," he warns before piercing my flesh. I scream as the liquid burns a path from the tumour site in my forearm to a network of lymph nodes in my armpit. It stings more than a little.

Now he banishes G to a chair across the room and presses a button. Inches from my body, white screens orbit me like satellite dishes. From an adjacent room, the radiologist sits in front of computer screens with the technician and resident doctor, watching as the dye blazes a trail through my body in real time.

There's more to do—more imaging tests, some bloodwork—and then I'm on the fourth floor, awaiting surgery in a rigid hospital bed. There are two other patients ahead of me, so we've got time to kill. I finish an article on my laptop while G answers emails on her phone. Finally, a middle-aged nurse with lime-green glasses comes over to offer me a heated blanket and, apparently, some comfort. "This must be really hard on you," she says, laying the blanket over my legs. "But at least your mom's here."

For a fleeting moment, I actually feel embarrassed for her. Until I don't.

"Uh, no. That's definitely not my mom."

"What … ?"

"This is my *wife*. And she's five years older than I am."

As the realization hits, her face falls. She scans her brain for a comeback. "It's ... it's just that you look so *young*," she says. "Which is *good!* You're lucky!"

But my irritation has nothing to do with vanity and everything to do with her assumption: this is an ugly case of heteronormativity. Refusing to consider that we might be queer, this nurse reached into her brain for the closest heterosexual explanation for the intimacy between us, picking—for whatever reason—'mother and daughter.' We are clearly close in age and don't look alike, yet she'd stuffed us into a box that obviously didn't fit. Even in an era of same-sex marriage, rainbow families, and out-and-proud celebrities, it's still the case that everyone is presumed straight (*innocent*) until proven gay (*guilty*).

As much as I hate being invisible now, I began my adult life content to hide in plain sight. As a cisgender woman with curly hair and curvy hips, I could pass quite easily. As a teen, I dated boys. No one questioned how much I loved Lilith Fair or painting naked women.

Many baby-dyke steps later, I came out of the closet and was no longer interested in hiding in plain sight. Now I wanted, quite desperately, for others to recognize me as queer—after all, how else would I find love (or sex)? But it wasn't happening. A classic femme problem, of course. To remedy this, I went online, signing up for a dating website where I eventually met my wife.

But I still craved visibility. Waitresses assumed that G and I were sisters. Tour guides assumed that we were BFFs. More than one of my clients thought "partner" was a business reference, not a romantic one. I grew tired of correcting assumptions and coming out, over and over and over again.

For years, I tried not to get my hackles up. *Some people just haven't been exposed to queers. This is a teaching opportunity*, I'd think. Somehow I'd explain away the ignorance. But as my health and life circumstances have become more complicated, this has changed. I find myself dealing with ignorance from health care professionals (doctors, nurses, psychologists, psychiatrists, dentists, chiropractors, etc.) during times of distress, when I really need to be understood and supported. My patience, as a queer patient, has grown as thin as the one-ply toilet paper in a clinic washroom.

Wearing only a paper gown and socks, I dangle my legs over the examination table as I wait. Finally, a knock, and Dr. B appears in her usual white lab coat. She's a middle-aged woman with black curly hair always cut short, and olive skin. Ever pleasant but never particularly warm, even after a few years of knowing me. But because family doctors are scarce—especially women—I'd stayed.

"How are you," she says. It is a statement, not a question.

"Good," I say, efficiently.

She quickly skims my file before moving on to the exam: checking eyes and ears, listening to heart and lungs, palpating stomach and kneading breasts. And lastly, the awkward business of a pap test.

When it's all over, she asks: "Anything else?" I swallow hard. This is a conversation I've been dreading for weeks.

"Actually, yes. My partner and I have decided to start a family."

Dr. B looks down at the chart. "But you're a lesbian, right?"

"Well, yeah. My partner is a woman."

"Okay. Then what's your plan?"

I take a breath. Clearly, if my partner were a man shooting blanks, she wouldn't be asking *me* for the solution.

"I guess I'd like a referral to the fertility clinic," I say.

"Why would you assume you're infertile?"

"I don't. But can't they order sperm there?"

She thinks a minute, tapping a pen against the clipboard. "Well, maybe.

But I don't think they treat lesbians."

It takes me a second to process what she's said.

"*Wait. What?*"

"I'm not sure they'd treat you."

"How can they *not* treat me? Wouldn't that be illegal?"

She nods, thoughtfully. "Hmm. That's a good question."

It *isn't* a good question: it's a rhetorical one. Of course they can't refuse to treat same-sex couples! This is Canada. This is 2010. We have a public health care system and same-sex marriage has been legal since 2005. I am an equal person under the law, aren't I?

In hindsight, I shouldn't have been shocked. This was the same doctor who'd been super confused a year earlier when I'd complained of pain during sex. I'd had to explain that sex between women could involve penetration, not just oral pleasure. Like a queer version of the birds-and-the-bees talk most of us get from our parents. In fact, just like a parent, I felt awkward as hell; but unlike a parent, I wished she'd just looked it up on the internet, for shit's sake.

Months later, I'm in a yoga class when the pain becomes too much to bear. I roll up my mat in a hurry and sprint across the parking lot to my vehicle, in tears. What began as a nagging pain in a back molar had become an abscess requiring a root canal. A second root canal would follow, a month later.

I resist coming out to the dentist, even though I am logging endless hours in his adjustable vinyl chair, wearing big plastic goggles that leave red rings around my eyes. There's far too much talk of church picnics and charity drives while I'm reclined with his gloved hands in my mouth. I can't tell if he's a queer-loving Unitarian or a fire-and-brimstone Baptist. To be safe, I refer to G as my "partner" and play the pronoun game. But I figure my health insurance card will eventually do the coming out for me, since it has my wife's first and last name on it.

Five years later, I am settling up my bill after a routine exam, when the receptionist asks, "What's your husband's full name again?"

This is a woman who has come to know me by name over the years. When I'm at the clinic, she tells me about the jewelry she's been making and weddings she's going to; I share stories about my busy toddler. And she still doesn't realize I'm queer?

"Um, I don't have a husband. Do you mean my partner, G?" I say.

She's silent for a moment as she squints at the computer screen: "Uh oh." It turns out that all of these years, she's been masculinizing my partner's name by switching her first name (a traditional woman's name) with her surname (a relatively common first name for a man). Miraculously, our insurance company had been correcting the error and compensating us anyway.

"I'm so sorry," says the receptionist. But she's apologizing for the mistake —not the assumption.

Months after I get pregnant, G and I travel to South Africa to visit my father. Our visit takes a dark turn when I begin bleeding on Christmas Day; by Boxing Day, I'm clearly miscarrying and the pain is horrible. Finally, the three of us drive to a hospital in Durban, just before midnight.

In the emergency room, I sit in an orange bucket chair—forehead to my knees—listening to the voices around me. I look up as a couple of triage nurses approach us.

"You're her husband?" says the man to my dad.

"Father."

"And where is her husband?" says the woman sweetly.

A hideous silence follows. I wait for G to break it, but she doesn't.

"Oh. Okay, okay. *No husband*. And you're her sister?" asks the woman.

My father tries to explain that she's my partner—not sister—but the message doesn't seem to stick. *Partner? What does that mean, exactly? This* is clearly a very North American term. Mid-conversation, I'm led away by a kind nurse in a burgundy uniform, looking a bit like a 1960s flight attendant. In an examination room, she gives me a shot of Demerol. It kicks in almost immediately.

The doctor comes in minutes later wearing a similar uniform and gold earrings that jangle as she walks. She puts a perfectly manicured hand on my shoulder and says: "This is such a painful thing, not just physically but psychologically." Because kindness makes me cry, I burst into tears. Because she isn't a Canadian doctor, she leans in for a hug and I accept it, with gratitude.

"This is difficult to ask," she says, releasing me. "But I take it this was an unwanted pregnancy?"

"Oh. Oh, no! Not at all," I say. For several minutes, I ramble on about being from Canada and wanting the baby with my whole heart. I can't find the words to say I'm a queer lady starting a family with my wife.

"But, no husband?"

"Well ... no," I say.

As she pats my shoulder—brown eyes overflowing with sympathy for the poor unmarried woman who'd gotten herself in trouble—I cry even harder.

I try to cut the South African doctor some slack. She treated me with more kindness than any Canadian doctor ever had, even if her narrative was all kinds of wrong. Somehow, I felt seen in spite of being othered. And in a place like South Africa, where same-sex marriage is legal but homosexuality is still condemned, the doctor may not have encountered any openly queer folks. These aren't excuses, just explanations. Maybe I'd be angry if I lived there.

But in my part of the world, there are neither good excuses nor compelling explanations. In Canada and the US, where the gay rights movement has had more traction, a lack of awareness boils down to willful ignorance or even contempt for the LGBTQ community. It feels particularly hostile coming from health care professionals who inevitably treat sexual and gender minority patients, whether they realize it or not. If doctors really are committed to the Hippocratic oath and trying to do no harm, a bit of education is in their best interests, too.

With ongoing health concerns, I'll continue to see more health care providers than I want to, many of whom will be shockingly ignorant. But, like a large metal syringe filled with blue radioactive dye, I'll keep poking holes in their heteronormative assumptions—even if it stings.

Sexualcentric institutions, ranging from the discipline of formal psychology to local medical clinics, may try to pathologize individuals who don't conform to their sexual assumptions, instead of recognizing pathology in their own policies, language, and structural organization. This can make asexuals reluctant to seek health services and can decrease those services' benefit to asexuals.

REMEDIAL ASEXUALITY

Sexualnormativity in Health Care

A. K. Morrissey

She, xe, and I sat on a park bench. "You had a panic attack and were writhing on the floor for two hours?" xe asked her.

"It's been happening once or twice a day for the past three months. I'm so overwhelmed with everything right now," she went on. "I can't control it."

"I think you need some professional help ..." xe trailed off as I frowned.

"Yeah," she snapped, "that usually works great for asexuals. I may as well be like, 'Hi, it'd be great if you could help me overcome my repression, give me a few sex tips, and maybe throw in some medication to increase my libido!'"

I wish I could say that exchange was an outlier, but it wasn't the first or last time I dealt with such considerations for others or myself. Asexuals sometimes make health care decisions—where to go, how to describe their medical history, if it's safe to subject themselves to professionals with institutional power to declare someone's perception of reality legally invalid and forcibly detain them—based on worry about their non-sexualness potentially being used as grounds for official (not to mention unofficial) pathologization of their minds and bodies.

Until the 2013 publication of the *Diagnostic and Statistical Manual of*

Mental Disorders (*DSM-V*), the American Psychological Association didn't formally acknowledge asexuality as an orientation differentiated from dysfunction. I've heard a wide variety of people rationalize the *DSM*'s prior treatment of non-sexualness by pointing out that distress and difficulty for a patient would be a necessary condition for a pathologizing diagnosis. Based on my own experiences as an asexual, I think this rationalization overlooks possible coercive pressures in diagnoses and/or treatment. Not that the manual's acknowledgment of asexuality necessarily precludes such coercion. And on top of that, it can simply be tough on a daily level to live a marginalized mode of existence without distress and difficulty. In my case, this struggle has been compounded by experiences with poverty, disability, and nonbinary trans identification. At the same time, factors such as my white privilege have in some ways mitigated my precarities.

Disclosure of asexual identity and/or practice to health professionals can be risky. Sometimes responses completely derail a conversation, suspicion and incredulity diverting energy away from more helpful inquiries. Though I don't claim to speak for all asexuals, I will say that such risks can make us hesitant to have discussions incorporating both our asexuality and our health problems for fear any issues will be misattributed to sexual dysfunction.

Asexuals with trauma symptoms risk having them leveraged by health care workers and others as evidence of the pathology of asexuality. This can particularly be the case with any symptoms an asexual considers a result of sexualcentric/sexualnormative oppression, whether they include anxiety, depression, nausea, panic attacks, or others. (By "sexualnormativity," in its simplest form, I mean the assumption that all people are sexual. I use "sexualcentricity" to refer to the closely related pervasive prioritization of sexualness and sexual relationships without adequate consideration of asexual ways of being.) Sexualcentric institutions, ranging from the discipline of formal psychology to local medical clinics, may try to pathologize individuals who don't conform to their sexual assumptions, instead of recognizing pathology in their own policies, language, and structural organization. This can make asexuals reluctant to seek health services and can decrease those services' benefit to asexuals.

I don't mean to imply asexuals never have positive experiences with health professionals. Still, I find it important to consider how some asexuals find themselves in a dilemma. Sexual-patriarchal relational systems overwhelm, from media glorifying sexual connection above other forms of intimacy and interaction, to medical, economic, and legal structures that automatically privilege sexual/domestic/romantic dyadic partnerships and genetic family bonds over other chosen platonic relationships and support systems. Oppressive social structures and micro-aggressive interpersonal interactions constantly grate on us, damaging our health and maybe even pushing us to seek care, but often available formal assistance is part of the same harmful system and populated by the same privileged persons.

Though care specifically designed for gender/sexual minorities may be better for asexuals than general care (often heteronormative by default), it can be just as sexualnormative. This can manifest itself in many ways depending on the care provider and the individual asexual, including the assumption that a patient is or wants to be partnered; being subconsciously or consciously less friendly with someone who doesn't engage in casual conversations about sexual attraction; not having resources that affirm asexual trans people imagining their transitioning/transitioned bodies in nonsexual ways; being complicit in insurance systems that disadvantage unconventional relational structures; and not believing a patient who insists they're not sexually active (even pushing a patient to undergo and pay for unnecessary procedures, such as testing to "rule out" the possibility that an apparent yeast infection is an STI, or exams like Pap smears that usually wouldn't be relevant to someone not sexually active with others). When seeking out resources specifically for gender/sexual minorities, I've sometimes concealed my asexuality by self-labeling as simply "queer"[1] to lessen my risk of being harassed or turned away. Entering those "safe" spaces can feel bittersweet.

To me, situations like that point to the importance of considering how an identity grouping that's in some ways "home" for someone can also be inhospitable for that person when dominated by group members who are privileged along other axes of identity, as scholar Kimberlé Crenshaw identified when coining "intersectionality." I see these dynamics at work when asexuals have to participate in erasure of our own asexuality in order to access needed resources. The home we sometimes find among gender/sexual minorities in general can be unsafe due to other gender/sexual minorities' sexual privilege.

Gender/sexual minorities' work toward mainstream medical and social acceptance raises complex questions about intersectionality and privilege. Prior to the *DSM*'s acknowledgment of asexuality, I would be conflicted when some lesbian and gay speakers would assert the validity of their identities through reference to past formal depathologization of homosexuality. Though asexuals have in certain ways recently been nominally admitted to that "club," I remain conflicted about how prominently institutions figure into many gender/sexual minorities' claims to legitimacy and safety. While that can be strategically pragmatic, I find myself dwelling on how dangerous Eurocentric psychology and medicine have been, and continue to be, for many minoritized groups. I'm not trying to disregard the work of gender/sexual minority activists who struggled for recognition—and those who still struggle. Acknowledgment can be particularly significant for people like asexuals, whose existence is threatened by erasure and/or conflation with other concepts like celibacy, sickness, or their social status. Nominal

1 Some asexuals consider asexuality queer and some don't, but that's a different discussion.

incorporation of asexuality, however, doesn't necessarily lead to a disruption of sexualcentric/sexualnormative institutions or guarantee that organizations, professionals, or society will be sensitive to asexuals or respectful of their needs.

Once, when I explained to an (alleged) ally how the *DSM*'s lack of acknowledgment of asexuality as an identity/orientation could be dangerous for asexuals on a practical level, he replied in an affronted and dismissive tone of voice, "Well, I've been diagnosed with chronic depression so I'm mentally ill too."

I stared, stunned that he didn't understand the difference between being diagnosed with depression and having what one might consider one's sexual orientation be pathologized. Not that depression isn't serious or that stigmatization of people diagnosed with mental illnesses isn't problematic. Rather, I see this exchange as a question of privilege. It seems his privileges contributed to his lack of awareness of the significance of our difference.

At the same time, based on my own experiences with disability, I can't help but think of the complicated relationship between asexual activism and disability activism. The prevalence of asexuals being involuntarily labeled as sick or disabled, and people with disabilities being involuntarily desexualized, and both being dehumanized, makes for complex conflicts and coalitional potentials. This can be especially true for people who find themselves in the intersections of these movements and identities. These precedents weigh heavily on us as we seek health care.

With the onset of my mobility-restricting and chronically painful physical condition having been exacerbated by socioeconomic factors preventing me from accessing adequate medical care, as well as by complications related to my nonbinary gender identity, I'm left wondering about a theoretical future when I might not have to choose between things like pursuing medical/technological options related to my disability and deliberating how best to survive the costs (financial, psychological, and social) of living in a trans body. In addition to that, I'm acutely aware that asexuals' gender identities (trans/gender-variant or not) are often held suspect on account of their asexuality. And I say that as someone with the privileges that come with having been medically read as normatively dyadic by birth, yet also as someone without a "masculine" vector in my subsequent transition away from attempting girl/woman performativities.

At the intersections of my crippled and asexual marginalities, I find myself in some ways privileged along those very axes. Between my disability and asexuality, I have the privilege of my disability not being used as commonly as some to "invalidate" and/or "explain" my asexuality (as if a pathological factor or source should necessarily discredit a person's experience and/or political positioning anyway). My disability also doesn't have a precedent of being commonly used as justification for involuntary sterilization or medicated sexual sedation. But these difficulties continue to seriously complicate health care for many.

Departing from those axes, though, as someone with white privilege, I find myself at much less risk of forced sterilization/medication and desexualization overall. My white privilege also protects me from the disproportionate violence directed against queer and especially trans people of colour, whose femininity is targeted by racialized transmisogyny, whose masculinity is criminalized by the police, and whose nonbinary identities are assailed by white supremacist colonialism. These violences are part of the reason it can be both significant and complicated to treat asexual identity as a category of orientation akin to (other) sexual orientation categories. It's necessary to try to account for how ideas of non-sexualness have been used by white supremacy.

Scholar Ianna Hawkins Owen explains these dynamics in "On the Racialization of Asexuality," in which she looks at racist controlling images such as the "mammy" and the "jezebel" as well as recent portrayals of asexuals in media. She points out how the idea of non-sexualness is at times pathologized and idealized. In what might be a surprising turn, sometimes when asexuality is pathologized, it's not done for the sake of marginalizing it—especially when asexuality is represented by white asexuals. Instead, asexuals are implicitly invited "to rejoin the pursuit of idealized whiteness through hypothetical cures and rehabilitation."[2] This underlying racist logic relies on fabricating hypersexualized blackness as a contrast to whiteness. It also implies that asexuals fail to achieve an ideal of "civilized restraint" simply (ironically) because they don't have "the sex drive that whiteness aspires to restrain," so they are labeled as "curable."[3] This insidious twisting together of pathologization of asexuality and misinterpretation of asexuality as an ideal perpetuates racism and denies the realities of people who identify as asexual and/or who live non-sexual lives. Measures taken in support of asexuality by health care providers should be placed in context of what Owen calls "a larger political project aimed at abolishing the problem of sexuality as a handmaiden to racial domination."[4]

I think these collisions clearly illustrate the necessity of health care providers, asexuals, and gender/sexual minorities as a whole seeking to operate with intersectional understandings of pathology and asexuality that both attend to immediate relief/reform of current practices and envision long-term work toward dismantling/subverting entire oppressive systems. Intersectionality also points to how it can be useful, when negotiating groupings and identification, to think of categories as somewhat coalitional: the "asexual community" can be considered a coalition of asexuals of different

2 Ianna Hawkins Owen, "On the Racialization of Asexuality," in *Asexualities*, ed. Karli June Cerankowski and Megan Milks (New York: Routledge, 2014): 264.

3 Ibid., 266.

4 Ibid., 272.

racial identities and gender identities, etc.; the "trans community," likewise; the "queer community," likewise. At the same time, in pursuing this sort of intersectional approach it can be significant not to universally impose a coalitional framework, so as not to assume that all kinds of oppression work exactly the same way. I wouldn't necessarily want to think of everything that might be considered its different forms (racism, ableism, sexism, etc.) in neat, equivalent pieces; instead of movements, or facets of identity, being interchangeable variables, they inseparably intertwine. The practical implications of this for medical professionals and people working to build up gender/sexual minority communities are substantial. Otherwise, people sometimes forget that understanding about one (or more) axis of oppression doesn't guarantee transitive understanding of all others.

Some experiences of verbal dehumanization I've had are oddly blunt. There've been conversations in which explaining my asexuality (answering, for example, interrogation about various life decisions—though more specifically I'm aromantic and nonlibidinal as well) resulted in the other person replying, in apparent seriousness and disgust, "You're not human." Now, I assume they weren't making a literal biological conclusion about what species to which I may or may not belong—and this sort of micro-dehumanizing instance functions quite differently than structural sexism or racism—but such a statement hardly seems benign. Sexuality/sexualness is widely assumed to be a fundamental part of human subjecthood—an assumption that plays itself out beyond interpersonal rudeness. It's important not to neglect to consider how these instances relate to larger patterns and systems.

A quick internet search yields "asexual bingo" cards that asexuals have compiled of acephobic reactions in person and online (not specific to medical contexts). Sadly, even other gender/sexual minorities sometimes do these. Reactions include denial, condescension, invasive personal questions/

accusations, sexual propositions, threats of "corrective" sexual assault, death threats, physical violence, and actual assault/rape.

Of course, similar oppressive reactions are commonly experienced by other gender/sexual minorities as well. We gender/sexual minorities "fail" to be human by not being straight, not being sexual, not being normatively gendered. And additional intersecting factors, such as ability, race, and legal status, are further variously used against "us" and by "us."

Popular knowledge often assumes asexuals have never been at risk of anything resembling conversion therapy. While I'm not sure attempts to eradicate asexuality have functioned quite the same way as destructive practices levied against some other gender/sexual minorities, asexuals can still be at risk of compulsorily imposed medical and psychological treatment intended to correct their supposed problem. Some asexuals have stories of receiving unwanted medication intended to increase their libido (unsolicited hormone prescriptions being tragic from some trans perspectives) and even forcible institutionalization and therapy to promote more "pro-social" behaviour. Though asexuals have some quite particular struggles, our experiences aren't entirely unlike those of other gender/sexual minorities, and there's potential for banding together through what we do share.

It's necessary to examine health care issues around asexuality beyond exclusion and reparative/corrective pressures directed at a sexual minority. It's important to pursue intersectionally informed practices of care and allyhood that don't disregard how difference can "go all the way down" between individuals but also between overlapping communities and movements. Attempting to account for and be respectful of these complexities is a necessary component of remedying disparities in health and health care.

Asexuals are often trapped between being ignored and receiving toxic attention in contexts of Eurocentric psychological and medical practice. If care providers are to help asexuals in the fullness of our experiences and identities instead of having us suffer for our asexuality, serious attention to personal and systemic sexualcentricity and sexualnormativity cannot be neglected. This is an indispensable part of the remedy for asexuals to thrive as participants in and contributors to LGBTQIA communities.

My experience isn't unique. The few studies that have examined bisexual people's experiences with health care have shown that we report a number of negative experiences, including having our identity judged, dismissed, or treated as evidence of illness

FIVE THINGS PROVIDERS NEED TO KNOW ABOUT BISEXUAL PEOPLE

Margaret Robinson

I am a health researcher and a bisexual woman with a history of activism in lesbian, gay, bisexual, trans, and queer (LGBTQ) communities. I've been out as bisexual for over twenty years—at work, to my family and friends, on the internet, and in newspapers. But I'm often not out to my doctors. This isn't unusual. Among sexual minority groups, bisexuals are least likely to be out to our health care providers, and our rate of non-disclosure may be as high as 47 percent.[1]

My first negative experience with a health care provider occurred soon after I came out. As an undergraduate I went to my university's health centre to get treatment for a stress-related yeast infection. I asked the doctor if it could be spread to my girlfriend.

"I don't see how," he said, "unless you took a bath and then she took a bath in the same water." I wasn't sure the doctor understood what I meant by "girlfriend."

1 Emily Page, "Mental health services experiences of bisexual women and men: An empirical study," *Journal of Bisexuality* 3 (2004): 137-160..

"What about if we're having sex?" I asked.

I didn't get an answer. Instead, he leaned around the side of his desk and peered intently at my shoes. To see if they were bisexual shoes, maybe. Since then I've had a therapist ask voyeuristic questions and imply that my bisexuality was the root of my stress, and I've had clinic staff assume that my bisexual identity means I have sex with multiple partners and am at high risk for sexually transmitted infections. These experiences left me feeling powerless and angry, and they did nothing to reduce my stress.

My experience isn't unique. The few studies that have examined bisexual people's experiences with health care have shown that we report a number of negative experiences, including having our identity judged, dismissed, or treated as evidence of illness. And the more severe our mental health issues are, the more bias we may experience from providers. These findings shouldn't be surprising, considering that most providers get very little training on gay and lesbian issues, and none at all on bisexuality. So think of this essay as a very quick bi boot camp.

1. Bisexuality is authentic and distinct

Studies over the past twenty years have shown that more sexual minority women identify as bisexual than as lesbian. When it comes to men, the pattern is reversed; more men identify as gay than as bisexual. When attractions are measured, most people report being attracted to both men and women (sadly, these studies have ignored non-binary genders). But when people discuss sexual identity it's often in binary terms, as if straight and gay/lesbian covered the whole range of sexuality (e.g., gay/straight alliances in schools).

Providers of health services can help improve the health of bisexual people by accepting our identity in the same way they accept straight, gay, or lesbian identities. Unfortunately, when many of us seek medical services, we encounter biphobia (bias against bisexuals) or monosexism (the view that being straight, gay, or lesbian is superior to being bisexual). The Re:searching for LGBTQ Health team conducted focus groups with bisexual people and asked them about experiences with mental health care. One woman described encountering biphobia from her health provider:

> Just the fact that I was, you know, into guys and girls. And as soon as [the provider] found that out it was "Oh, I think that's disgusting." And I thought, okay, well, I can't trust any advice or anything you're going to give me if you're strongly disagreeing with my lifestyle. So I opted to no longer see her.[2]

Bisexual people can encounter biphobia even in service agencies designed to serve sexual minority people. Some of my most biphobic experiences have been with providers who serve the gay and lesbian community, or who identify as gay or lesbian themselves, which has been both frustrating and deeply disappointing.

Another issue was a tendency for providers to dismiss the authenticity of bisexual identity, and to pressure bisexual people to identify as straight or as gay/lesbian. As one man said, "I had one therapist say, 'Oh, well you just have to choose.'"[3] I've had providers make jokes about my identity, or suggest that I should only date men since "it's easier." Accepting bisexual identity as authentic will reduce the stress we face as bisexual people when accessing health services.

Bisexuality is an identity distinct from being straight, gay, or lesbian. However, information about bisexual health is difficult to find because until recently researchers tended to combine information from gay, lesbian, and bisexual people. As researchers learn how important it is to compare sexual

2 Allison Eady, Cheryl Dobinson, and Lori E. Ross, "Bisexual people's experiences with mental health services: A qualitative investigation," *Community Mental Health Journal* 47 (2011): 381.

3 Ibid., 382.

minority groups to one another (and not only to our straight peers), we've begun to realize that bisexual health can often look different than the health of gay, lesbian, or straight people.

2. Bisexual people experience stigma and stress

Bisexual people experience the same stressors as the general population, such as those related to work, family, or finances. Like gay and lesbian people, we also experience homophobic prejudice and heterosexist discrimination or violence, and may internalize homophobia, further damaging our health. In addition, bisexual people experience prejudice and discrimination related to our bisexual identity, such as biphobia and monosexism, and may internalize these as well. This means that bisexual people must cope with a heavy stress burden to remain healthy.

Since we also have other identities, such as gender, race, age, or class, we may experience intersecting stigma and discrimination. For example, I experience stigma as a bisexual, as a woman, and as an Indigenous Canadian, but also specifically as a two-spirit woman—an Indigenous woman who is a member of a sexual or gender minority. Womanist scholars and activists have noted that racial, gender, and sexuality stigma is not additive, but *interactive*, with additional stigmas actually multiplying stress. I may, for example, be more likely to experience biphobic or homophobic violence because I am Indigenous, and may be seen as an easier target with less social power.

Many bisexual people are also poor and experience financial stress. A California study found that bisexual women reported the highest rates of poverty (17.7 percent) of all sexual orientations, while poverty rates for bisexual men (9.7 percent) fell between those for straight men (who were the poorest) and those of gay men, who were the least poor.[4] In Canada, 34.9 percent of bisexual men and 42.7 percent of bisexual women fall into the bottom fifth of household income.[5] These high rates of poverty may be another case of intersecting oppression, with our incomes being impacted by our sexual identity and our gender, and possibly by issues such as the resources and support we have to pursue education.

Whatever the cause, stigma and stress have a negative impact on our health. Stress releases hormones that raise blood pressure and lower the immune system, initiate weight gain, and are associated with anxiety and depression. Due to the stress we face, bisexual people, especially women, have important health differences when compared to our gay, lesbian, and straight peers.

3. Bisexual people have significant health disparities

Many providers imagine that health disparities will fall on a continuum, with straight people experiencing the fewest health problems, gay/lesbian people experiencing the most, and bisexual people falling in the middle. But in many cases bisexuals experience the greatest health disparities. Among these, issues such as depression, anxiety, suicide, and substance use stand out. These issues are bisexual issues not because they result from having a bisexual identity, but because they result from experiences (such as discrimination) commonly experienced by bisexual people.

Depression and anxiety: Bisexual men and women consistently report significantly high levels of depression and anxiety compared to straight people.

4 Randy Albelda, M.V. Lee Badgett, Gary J. Gates and Alyssa Schneebaum, "Poverty in the lesbian, gay, and bisexual community," The Williams Institute (2009): 7. http://williamsinstitute.law.ucla.edu/wp-content/uploads/Albelda-Badgett-Schneebaum-Gates-LGB-Poverty-Report-March-2009.pdf

5 Michael Tjepkema, "Health care use among gay, lesbian and bisexual Canadians," Health Reports 19 (2008): 57.

A large US study found that participants attracted to both men and women had the highest rates of stress and depression.[6] In my country, Canada, over a quarter of bisexual women (25.2 percent) have a diagnosed mood disorder, such as depression, and 17.7 percent have a diagnosed anxiety disorder.[7] These rates are significantly higher than those for other women. For men, 11.4 percent have a diagnosed mood disorder, and 10.1 percent have a diagnosed anxiety disorder.[8] These rates are similar to those for gay men, but significantly higher than those for straight men.

Suicide: In many studies bisexual people report high levels of self-harm, suicide attempts, and thoughts of suicide. In a recent study, 18 percent of bisexual people reported thinking about suicide in the past year.[9] Such thoughts are more common among youth, with bisexuals age twenty-five and younger thinking about suicide at a significantly higher rate than bisexual people over age twenty-five.[10]

Substance use: One of the ways people attempt to cope with high levels of stress is to use substances, and bisexuals are no exception. A US study found that 54 percent of bisexual men used tobacco, compared with 40 percent of gay men.[11] Among bisexual women, 62 percent used tobacco, compared with 49

6 Lisa L. Lindley, Katrina M. Walsemann, and Jarvis W. Carter Jr., "The association of sexual orientation measures with young adults' health-related outcomes," *American Journal of Public Health* 102 (2012): 1177-85.

7 Tjepkema, "Health care use," 58.

8 Ibid.

9 Lori E. Ross, Greta R. Bauer, Melissa A. MacLeod, Margaret Robinson, Jenna MacKay, and Cheryl Dobinson, "Mental health and substance use among bisexual youth and non-youth in Ontario, Canada," Public Library of Science 1 (2014): e101604.

10 Ross, et al., "Mental health and substance use," e101604.

11 Joseph G.L. Lee, Adam O. Goldstein, Leah M. Ranney, Jeff Crist, and Anna McCullough, "High Tobacco Use among Lesbian, Gay, and Bisexual Populations in West Virginian Bars and Community Festivals," *International Journal Of Respiratory Public Health* 8 (2011): 2764.

percent of lesbian women.[12] In my home province of Ontario, 31.2 percent of bisexuals exhibit symptoms of problem drinking.[13]

The illegal substance used most frequently by bisexual people is cannabis. In the US National Alcohol Study, for example, 37.8 percent of bisexual women reported using cannabis within the past year, compared with 21.1 percent of lesbians and 5 percent of straight women.[14] In my own work, bisexual women report using cannabis to cope with anxiety and depression.[15] In a number of studies, bisexual women are most likely to report using cocaine, tranquilizers, hallucinogens, ecstasy, amphetamines, and heroin. However, while our rate of use for these drugs is higher than for other women, the percentage of bisexual women using them is extremely small.

Researchers tend to combine information on bisexual men with that of gay men, so we have far less information about bisexual men's health, including their substance use. Some studies show that bisexual men have high rates of amphetamine, tranquilizer, inhalant, and injection drug use, but again, while the rates are high, the percentage of men using these drugs is very small.

Some issues we face intersect with others. For example, bisexual women report high rates of violence throughout our lifetimes, and those of us who experience violence are more likely to use drugs or alcohol.

4. Bisexual People Lack Social Support

The support of family, friends, and communities makes it easier to cope with

12 Ibid.

13 Ross, et al., "Mental health and substance use," e101604.

14 Karen F. Trocki, Laurie A. Drabble, and Lorraine T. Midanik, "Tobacco, marijuana, and sensation seeking: Comparisons across gay, lesbian, bisexual, and heterosexual groups," *Psychology of Addictive Behaviors* 23 (2009): 620.

15 Margaret Robinson, "The Role of Anxiety in Bisexual Women's Use of Cannabis," *Psychology of Sexual Orientation and Gender Diversity* 2 (2015): 142.

stress, even if our stress levels are very high. Having someone to talk with us about our problems or to take care of us when we are sick improves our mental and physical health. However, many bisexual people lack this kind of social support in our daily lives. In a study that examined factors impacting the mental health of bisexual people, participants reported that partners, family members, friends, colleagues, and the LGBTQ community were often unsupportive of bisexuals and bisexual identity.[16] For example, one participant in their study reported, "My sister said to me … 'I would prefer it if you were just my gay brother, and not this slutty person who just sleeps with everyone.'"[17]

5. Our Health Can Improve

When we build a supportive network of friends, family, and community, our health gets better. Accessing health services can be part of that process. Bisexuals report good results with providers who have a positive attitude toward bisexuality, who ask open-ended questions, and who educate themselves about bisexuality.[18] Having providers respond positively to bisexuality makes it easier to come out in the future, and reduces the stress associated with coming out.

As a health researcher, I work to improve access to information about bisexual health, about the negative impact of stress, and the positive role of support. As a bisexual woman, I've seen the impact of stigma and stress in my own life and in the lives of people in my bisexual community. I want health care providers who understand the impact of biphobia and monosexism, and who can help us strategize healthy ways to cope. But since many bisexual health

16 Allison Eady, Cheryl Dobinson, and Lori E. Ross, "Perceived determinants of mental health for bisexual people: A qualitative examination," *American Journal of Public Health* 100 (2010): 499.

17 Ross et al., "Perceived determinants," 498.

18 Ibid., 383.

issues are the result of systemic injustice, I'd also like health care providers to oppose biphobia, monosexism, and other forms of discrimination when they see it. Because social justice is good for our health.

QUEER AND TRANS HEALTH INNOVATION PROFILE

The Affirmations Deck (Toronto, Ontario)

Carly Boyce,
Coordinator, Filling in the Blanks Project,
Planned Parenthood Toronto

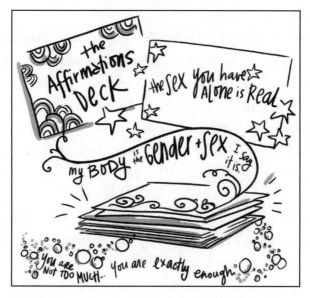

Tell us about the Affirmations Deck and why you're proud of it.

The Affirmations Deck contains sixty-two supportive statements meant to affirm the existence and experiences of queer and trans youth. It was created by a group of fourteen queer and/or trans youth volunteers through a queer sex education project at Planned Parenthood Toronto in 2014. Our project team thought about things we wished we had when we were struggling with our identities, or with the erasure, normativity, and violence in our everyday world. We couldn't gift everyone with good friends or families who would love them for exactly who they are, so we made these as a way to create supportive environments. When young people feel seen and valued, it affects how we see ourselves and our ability to create change in our lives and communities. We hope that this deck continues to find its way into the hands of young queer and trans folks who might not otherwise have access to supportive communities, the precise thing that keeps so many of us alive. These cards are a kiss we blew to our slightly younger selves, and to young people struggling with experiences of marginalization without folks who have their backs.

The cards have hand-drawn motifs on them that correspond to their subject matter, almost like suits in a deck of playing cards. They address topics like bodies, consent, gender, healing, self-love, and relationships. Folks can look at them when they need support, colour them in, hang them in their locker, carry them in their pocket, send them in the mail, or hide them in library books with queer subtext. They can be journaling prompts or workshop debriefing tools. They can be used and shared in lots of different ways! They are available as a free printable PDF as well as in hard copy from Planned Parenthood Toronto.

We don't know where the thousand or so decks that have been distributed so far have ended up, or how many folks have printed their own, but we do know that groups of youth are considering translating them into other languages and writing their own affirmations that speak to the particularities of their experiences. We also know that they have been sent to queer and trans people who are incarcerated, to therapists, acupuncturists, guidance counsellors, community health nurses, sex educators, and other folks who work with youth.

If someone from another place emailed you to say, "I want to do this in my community," and asked for your advice on how to do it, what would you tell them?

The hardest (but most fun) part of this process was finalizing our list of affirmations. We talked at length about whether cards should be written in the first or second person (we settled on a mix), and how to balance specificity with universality. For example, the card that reads *It's okay that you started that fight at a family gathering* started off as *It's okay that you yelled at your dad at thanksgiving.* We also struggled with affirming negative experiences, which led to cards like *I am truly sparkly and amazing when I am able to get what I need from an unjust medical system, It's not my fault that I have internalized my experiences of oppression,* and *My pronouns are not too complicated.*

Is there anything else you'd like to tell us?
My current favourite cards are *The sex you have alone is real, My relationships do not have to look the way I have been taught relationships should look,* and *You are not too much—you are exactly enough.*

For more information about the Affirmations Deck (and to download the deck!), visit pptto.tumblr.com/post/104932883080/ the-affirmations-deck-is-here

It's clear to us that looking at past differences and addressing stigma is so important, as well as loving and working with one another. This journey began and continues with self-reflection, honest conversations, and vulnerabilities.

BREAKING DOWN BARRIERS

A Journey to Increase Collaboration and Understanding Between LGBT2-SQ and Medical Communities

Jenna J. Webber and Rita O'Link

It is a tale as old as time: two people from different backgrounds, each a mystery to the other, find a way to connect with and understand one another despite the pressures and stigmas of the outside world. The way we see it, if this is true in so many popular stories, why can't medical, educational, and Lesbian, Gay, Bisexual, Transgender, Two-Spirited and Queer (LGBT2-SQ) communities and individuals work together with the common goal of better health for all? The answer: we can!

Over the past year we—Rita (an advocate and member of the trans community in Sudbury, Ontario), and Jenna (a medical student at the Northern Ontario School of Medicine, NOSM)—have embarked on a journey of breaking down barriers. Through this we have grown together with community and student members to create a solid foundation for understanding, respect, and collaboration between LGBT2-SQ and medical communities in Sudbury, a mining city of 160,000 people in Northern Ontario. This might sound like a grand and unattainable goal; it could have been if it was tackled alone. Instead, through collaboration, mutual respect, and trust, we were able to create an LGBT2-SQ handbook for health care providers as well as a proposed intake form, both of which use inclusive and informative language to promote understanding and safety.

To develop these resources, NOSM partnered with TgInnerselves, a trans advocacy group serving all of Northern Ontario, as well as Réseau ACCESS Network, an organization dedicated to harm and risk reduction, wellness, and education. Students from NOSM along with representatives from these organizations held focus group sessions with members of the LGBT2-SQ community, during which participants raised concerns and desires regarding their health care. The themes that arose most often were: safe and inclusive communication with health care professionals (inclusive of pamphlets, posters, advertisements, forms, and face-to-face interactions); consistent, dependable, and open collaboration between patients, general practitioners, and specialists; the use of inclusive and safe gender-neutral language in intake and personal forms; and respect for the privacy and autonomy of individuals in all matters of health, including the use of preferred names under specified circumstances. Once these themes were identified, focus group participants developed tips for health care professionals to make care more accessible, inviting, and safe in each of these domains, all of which are included in the handbook. Since its distribution, we have received great feedback from health care providers who tell us they now feel more comfortable asking questions relating to gender or sexual identity in a safe and appropriate way.

It's clear to us that looking at past differences and addressing stigma is so important, as well as loving and working with one another. This journey began and continues with self-reflection, honest conversations, and vulnerabilities. Let us share our own stories with you.

Jenna

I was born and raised in a Northern Ontario mining town, four generations deep into the gold veins, ore deposits, and birch trees that surround the region. With two loving and accepting parents, and a playfully torturous but fiercely loyal and supportive big brother, the world was mine to discover—as long as it didn't involve driving past sunset during moose season or exposing my midriff during my "delicate" teen years.

Although I loved my hometown and respected the lessons it taught me, my experiences growing up in a northern community made me aware at a young age of the stigmas and barriers to health care that some people face. I spent most of my life without a family doctor or local walk-in clinic, having to use the emergency room whenever a health issue arose. It was usually staffed by locums (visiting doctors); many were great, but some seemed far more concerned about the billing codes than me as a person. Often I didn't feel comfortable seeking care for even a sore stomach for fear of judgment. As a cisgendered, heterosexual female, I can't begin to imagine the fear I'd feel if I had to seek care saying, "Well, I was born a female but I've spent my whole life knowing deep inside that I'm a boy and I can't deny it anymore. Please help me." This is a fear that I hope my patients, their families, neighbours, and friends never experience. I hope they feel comfortable and accepted speaking about whatever thoughts, feelings, or troubles affect them.

You might be asking yourself how these reflections spurred a desire to partner with and advocate for LGBT2-SQ health and rights so many years later. In a general sense, I have always felt drawn to helping people and populations who experience marginalization as a result of social inequities. Meeting Rita for the first time provided me with inspiration, energy, and strength. It ignited a voice and fire within me, drawing me more certainly than ever to LGBT2-SQ health.

I first met Rita during a presentation we had organized with Vincent

Bolt and Darlyn Hansen of TgInnerselves in celebration of the Day of Pink, an annual event aimed at ending homophobic and transphobic bullying. Their honesty, vulnerability, strength, and vision inspired me. I contacted Rita with the basic idea for this project and it blossomed.

Throughout this journey, I have been consistently impressed by the honesty and vulnerability that individuals shared with us. The simple question, "How can we help?" incited people to expose interactions and fears that they might not have shared with others. They told us painful yet heartwarming stories that were full of emotion and lessons to be learned by all, no matter their profession. There was one particular moment in which this vulnerability became painfully obvious to me.

I was driving from my hometown some three-and-a-half hours north of Sudbury to a focus group session and was running late. I could feel a tension rising in my chest as I thought, *Oh my goodness, I showered last night, not today. My hair is a mess and I can't show up without makeup. That would be unprofessional.* It took me a few moments to realize the hypocrisy in what I was saying. I was shocked and frankly disappointed in myself that I would ask others to share their vulnerabilities with me and applaud them for their courage, but I wouldn't show up sans cover-up or mascara. I thought about Rita in this moment, who would not have looked at me any differently if I had shown up in a red-carpet-worthy ball gown or yesterday's work boots and gardening clothes. It was an important lesson in perspective and walking-the-walk.

I feel incredibly blessed and honoured to have the time and teachings from Rita, her peers, and all focus group participants. This project, and this journey, has made me a better person, and I thank Rita from the bottom of my heart. Looking forward, I am excited and inspired as we continue to work together with the goal of bettering trans health care across the North. Watch out, society: we've got more passion than a drugstore paperback novel and we're just getting started.

Rita

Sixty-one years of age now ... It has been a long road. I ran from what I am for decades. I tried the hyper masculinity thing. I tried religion. I tried whatever I could but found I was unable to make it go away or to outrun it. About eight years ago I could no longer run; I was just too tired. I turned to face what I am and took the daring chance: to accept the truth of my self and try to see if there was any good to be found in what I am. I came out to my family, close friends, church, and business clients. This I will tell you: Mount Everest is a speed bump in a parking lot compared to that climb. I still don't know how I did it and I'm still dealing with severe familial repercussions.

The climb out of self-loathing, depression, and self-worthlessness is a monumental, soul-draining challenge that is and always will be a work-in-progress. It is hard work being me ... so be it ... onwards ... Freedom ... freedom to breathe ... freedom to step out into the everyday world and just take my place along with everyone else ... that's all I wanted and all I want now ... but how do you do that when your physical body says one thing and your heart says another? How does one transition? What is transition, anyway?

I sought out a therapist to help me. The questions: What am I? How can I be sure? There are no answers from without ... absolute surety is an illusion. I have to work to be me ... especially with a body that screams that I am not. My therapist never answered my questions directly; always let me come to my own conclusions. Together we cleared away the debris so that I could see for myself, so I could see who I was. I never sought HRT (Hormone Replacement Therapy) or SRS (Sex Reassignment Surgery). These were things too far for me ... things too scary to contemplate. My therapist was so patient; she let me take my time, to make those decisions myself when I was ready. When I eventually did ask her for a referral letter for HRT, I also asked her if she thought I was ready. Her reply was that I was ready almost two years earlier.

In the midst of all this self-discovery, I became an activist, quite by accident. I knew my struggle and saw the incredible struggle of others. I couldn't remain silent ... I had to speak out, combining this need with the search for a doctor who would help me with HRT that led me to the doors of the Northern Ontario School of Medicine. But I couldn't find any doctor who would help. They were either uncomfortable with the concept, or felt they didn't have the right training ... all understandable, but it left me feeling desperate. What is far worse than no treatment available is when a treatment *is* available but denied. Despair in full measure ... overflowing, not just for me, but also for so many like me ...

The primary purpose of HRT is not for the physical changes that it causes, though those changes are also extremely important as we struggle to get our bodies more in line with our hearts; it is for our brain. This I will tell you: running your brain on the wrong hormones is hell; nothing is ever right. Until the mind is right, the rest of one's life never will be. Finally, after four-and-a-half years, I found a doctor willing to help—and that doctor is a graduate of NOSM! Finally some relief ... finally some desperately needed help ... but just for me. And that is not enough.

One day I was part of a group from TgInnerselves that was invited to NOSM to present during their Day of Pink—a chance to engage and implore for help from the up-and-coming medical community. I met Jenna there, and so many more. It would seem that our words got through and were inspiring. I needed to make it easier for others like me, those who perhaps were not blessed with the red hair and yakky personality that I have been given. I needed to speak up for those who could not speak up for themselves. The fire was lit and the response has been overwhelming. A number of initiatives have been launched to improve the education and practice of medical treatment for trans persons here in Northern Ontario. This is groundbreaking and so very exciting! We have new LGBT2-SQ curriculum modules being developed for both the undergraduate and the graduate programs. We have a new inclusive LGBT2-SQ patient form that will be given to all patients. There is also a doctor/patient question list and approach to help with the one-on-one interviews.

The world is changing, and that change is happening right here. And we are all part of that change ... working together ... heart to heart ... making a desperately needed difference in the lives of real people.

What's Next for Us

So, the logical question: what next? We have had an incredible journey building strong friendships and collaborations to break down barriers for our local LGBT2-SQ peoples. Now we hope to extend our borders to all of Northern Ontario and other rural and remote areas of the country. In March 2016 we presented a workshop based on our collaboration at the Rainbow Health Ontario national LGBT2-SQ health conference, and have successfully distributed our health care provider handbook across the country via the Rainbow Health Ontario website. The handbook was also featured at the first Trans Health Conference for the North, from the North, an event we helped to co-organize in April 2016 to educate professionals on the provision of safe and inclusive health care for all and to create opportunities for collaboration across Northern Ontario. We are aiming to have the handbook translated into French, and are open to other initiatives that will enable us to increase accessibility and safety for all patients.

We recognize the unique health care challenges and triumphs faced by those living in rural and remote areas, and it is our mission to ensure that everyone, no matter their geographic status, has access to help and support, both medically and socially, when they want and need it. Rita and I are only two people, but by reaching out, educating, and engaging others, we hope to create champions in LGBT2-SQ health and health care across Canada.

We encourage and urge you to take up this task in any way you can, so that we may finally experience safe, equitable, and appropriate health care for all.

The OB turned out to be lovely, actually trans competent, and queer. He was less interested than my midwife was in me having a C-section, willing to let me stay pregnant longer, better at informed consent, and a far better listener. By the end of my first visit with the OB, I liked him better than the midwife, trusted him more, and felt better supported ... Everyone I knew had prepared me to love midwives and be cautious around OBs— meeting Mark Yudin was my first lesson in specificity. Who your care providers are matters far more than their role or professional training.

BABY ESCAPE PLAN TWO

j wallace skelton

We had a baby. Which is simultaneously the most ordinary thing, and an absolute miracle. UNICEF says that 353,000 babies are born every day, which makes birth an event I am sharing with more people than I can imagine, mundane and common. Yet in my life, this is magical, miraculous— the sudden appearance of a new person who never before existed, and who needs me in a particular urgent way. Birth is never just one thing.

The story begins well before birth though. I'm a trans guy who still has all original parts. I'm partnered to another trans guy, and we conceived, as they say, with a little help from our friends. There were visits to fertility clinics for cycle monitoring, trips to see the spunkle, and lots of hoping and wishing.

While the pee stick from the first positive pregnancy test was still wet, I called the local midwives. I wanted midwifery care because I wanted to know the providers who would be at the birth. I wanted to make sure that by then, they would get my name right, my pronouns right, and talk about my body in language that felt comfortable to me. I wanted midwives so that I could give birth at home, in a space I could control, where I would not become some sort of trans curiosity. I wanted midwives because as a trans guy, birth made me feel vulnerable, and I needed advocates I could trust to work with me and support me.

I got lucky with that first pregnancy. The midwives consistently used my name (not my legal name), always referred to me as he/him, called other care providers if they had to make a referral and made sure they would get things right, and required all the staff in labour and delivery at the local hospital to have trans competency training even though the hospital was just our back-up plan. And when the baby preferred the back-up plan to the birth-at-home plan, they arranged for me to have a private room at the hospital, and made sure there was an appropriate sign on the door and information in my chart. I could not have wished for better.

So the second time I got a positive pregnancy test, in a different city five years later, I again contacted midwifery practices looking for care. Then I had to call them back to say that this pregnancy was not going to result in a baby. Some months after, again with a slightly damp pee stick in hand, I contacted local midwifery clinics. And then eight weeks later, I again miscarried and had to tell them I no longer needed midwifery care. Exactly a month after that, with the next positive pee stick, I was more hesitant, but I called and was offered initial appointments at two practices. When the time came and I was still pregnant, my partner and I met and interviewed two midwives. While neither felt great, meeting with two felt like having a choice, and we went with the one who actually asked how I was feeling.

We left that first appointment telling ourselves that we could not expect this midwife to be as perfect as the first ones, and assumed that we would warm to each other with time. She knew that trans people existed and seemed to care about how I was doing. We settled into a rhythm. At each visit, I noticed that she was still using my legal name in my file and I talked to her about how inappropriate that was, and repeated my name. She'd nod, and say that she'd make the changes, but at the next appointment we'd do the whole dance over again. She was otherwise careful about the trans thing, but it was as if she was so careful about the trans thing she forgot other aspects of care. Tests were conducted late. Referrals were late. It always felt like there was an air of panic and decisions had to be made right away because we were running out of time. She promised that she would be there for the birth, but the way she said it indicated that it wasn't about me, but more like a badge of honour for her, as if she wanted to be able to say that she had a trans client and had delivered his baby. Except she didn't want me to deliver my baby, she wanted me to have a scheduled C-section at exactly forty weeks gestation. At the time, it seemed odd that a midwife would push for a C-section, but I took the referral to the OB, because hey, that baby had to come out somehow. Now I wonder if she wanted me to have a C-section because that way she would never have to see, touch, or talk about my genitals. She could say she was the trans guy's midwife and never have to look at my actual trans body.

The OB turned out to be lovely, actually trans competent, and queer. He was less interested than my midwife was in me having a C-section, willing to let me stay pregnant longer, better at informed consent, and a far better listener. By the end of my first visit with the OB, I liked him better than the midwife, trusted him more, and felt better supported. I absolutely left my first meeting with him feeling better, and for the first time, hopeful about this birth. Everyone I knew had prepared me to love midwives and be cautious around OBs—meeting Mark Yudin was my first lesson in specificity. Who your care providers are matters far more than their role or professional training. Mark thought it would be okay for me to stay pregnant longer, so I had a few more days to try and go into labour. I booked a C-section with him for forty weeks and five days, as the back-up plan.

Our last visit with the midwife was at thirty-eight weeks. This was the first appointment where I did not initiate the conversation about how

I needed her to use my actual name. At the time in the visit where I would usually explain that it was not appropriate and not legal to continue to use my birth name when I had so clearly explained that I never used it, she launched the conversation instead. She explained that she had been sent a video clip of my husband on CBC talking about how "deadnaming" trans people is inappropriate. She said she finally understood why calling me by my actual name was so important and that she would get it right from now on. I decided that if it took thirty-eight weeks and a spot on national TV for her to understand what my husband was saying (although still not what I was saying), this was not going to work. At thirty-eight and a bit weeks pregnant, we fired our midwife.

We spilled our frustrations to Jay Macgillvray, another midwife, one we knew and respected. She listened, said that she thought "community should really look after community" and that she knew someone she thought might be able to help. She made a phone call, and delivered us to midwife number two.

Midwife two, Jen Goldberg, was a different deal entirely. I didn't have to edit the intake forms—her practice already used language that acknowledged that *people* can be pregnant, not just women. Jen instructed us to write a birth plan and asked us detailed questions about what we wanted. She offered suggestions, answered questions, and explained processes and procedures in detail. She made sure that the hospital knew a trans guy would be having a baby there, included information about trans people in our chart, and ensured that the hospital provided trans competency training to staff in labour and delivery and post-partum care. Instead of pushing me to have a C-section, she asked if that was really what I wanted. When the most compelling statement I could make was that I had a C-section booked, she asked again what I wanted. And then she checked in. I finally admitted that it wasn't what I wanted, but I'd made an appointment and unless I could manage to go into labour first, I thought I should do what I agreed I would do. She reminded me I could cancel it, but I pressed on anyway.

On the morning of the scheduled C-section, we rose early. I walked to the hospital. It felt like the only part of the birth that I could do myself, and I was not going to hand that over to a taxi driver. Secretly I hoped that the vigorous walk with luggage would get labour started. It didn't. We checked in. The staff were positive, warm, and welcoming. I was grim and resistant. Sabrina, the friendly nurse assigned to prep me for surgery, asked if I was ready to meet my baby, and I said something surly back. She closed the door and said, "You know, nobody can force you to have a C-section."

Sometimes a single statement makes all the difference. Her words allowed me to say no, to ask about other options. By the time Jen arrived, the conversation was no longer about a possible C-section, but was instead about induction. Nobody, not even the OB, pressured me to have the C-section. Jen checked to make sure there was no medical reason the baby had to be born that morning, and helped us schedule an induction for two days later. We took a cab home from the hospital and had a very awkward conversation with our five-year-old about where exactly his long awaited baby sibling was.

My body had two more days to work on getting ready. By the morning of our scheduled induction (baby escape plan two), I was having regular contractions. This time, I agreed to take a cab to the hospital. This time, right from the beginning I got to say yes or no every step of the way. Knowing my concern about students and other people coming to ogle me, Jen controlled who came in and out of our room. She tracked down nurses and doctors she trusted for procedures, barred people from entry, and set the tone when other care providers did come in, modeling the right language for me and my body. Jen made sure I knew what was going to happen, that I had a chance to not only to ask questions, but also to say yes or no.

At the very end of the day, just before the baby was born, Jen said to my husband, "Bear, come catch your baby." And then again, a little more urgently, because the time was upon us, "Bear, come catch your baby!" And he did. I launched the baby, and my husband caught him. Jen made the space for that, protected it, respected us, required others to respect us or step away, and in doing so, allowed this to be about us and our family. We had a baby, and it was magic.

The way I was treated in the ER—the misgendering, deadnaming, ignorance, and the lack of discretion I experienced—is incredibly dangerous. When I say it was "my last visit," I mean it. I will not voluntarily return to an ER the next time I'm feeling suicidal. Anything would be a better option than experiencing that level of embarrassment and shame again. Embarrassment and shame, from those who were meant to take care of me.

MIND YOUR WORDS

Xeph Kalma

I want to kill myself. Badly. I don't know if it's because of the instinct to survive or what, but I get myself to an emergency room. I'm having another extreme bout of depression brought on by gender dysphoria. As a trans woman who has lived with depression her entire life, this is something that happens on the regular for me. And if I can't be transferred into a crisis unit tonight, get the help I so desperately need, and make it through the next few days, this will probably happen again.

So, here I am. Lying on a bed in the emergency room, momentarily happy that I'm safe and that the people here are trained to take care of me. I put my trust in them, because I can't trust myself. It's not easy to do. To surrender my autonomy. To admit that I'm failing. To tell a total stranger, "Hey, I feel like I might kill myself if I'm left alone right now, and I need some help." It's risky, because you might end up being held for a day, three days, three weeks, or more. It's risky, because if the people who are meant to take care of you don't know how to do that properly, you may end up leaving feeling worse and more lost than before.

During the patient intake process, I attempted to make it very clear which pronouns were the correct ones to use when talking to or about me. This is my first visit to the hospital after having the gender marker on my health card corrected, so I'm very optimistic that it will go better than others in the past. There were little Fs (for "female") all over the place: in the hospital documents, on my wristband, and on my chart. This made me pretty happy. That happiness was crushed when I left the waiting room and entered the emergency room. It only takes minutes for me to realize that whatever is on my chart will be trumped by my appearance—the very same appearance that causes me dysphoria, the very same appearance that is a major contributing factor to me being in the ER to begin with. Unbeknownst to the staff in that ER, by calling me "he" and "him," they have all become a grim reminder of exactly why I'm here.

My deadname, that other dysphoria-spewing beast, is also going to be a problem. A deadname is a name from the past that no longer applies to a trans person if they decided to choose their own name. Deadnames can be a painful reminder of a terrible time in a person's life. They are tenacious and require resources to fix legally, which many trans folx do not have. Because of this, mine still exists in the legal sense. In an attempt to counter this during the intake process, I tried to make it abundantly clear that even though my deadname might show up on some files, it is not in fact my name and is certainly not how I want to be addressed, especially while in a suicidal state of mind. This tactic has worked in the past, but today, the message either isn't passed along to the staff treating me or else is simply ignored.

I'm repeatedly deadnamed, leaving me feeling worse than when I arrived at the hospital. It makes me wonder why I even sought help here in the first place.

While being asked questions about my health, I am asked what medications I'm currently taking. Since I've chosen to go down the HRT route, I tell the hospital staff that I'm on a testosterone blocker (formerly spironolactone), as well as estradiol. The nurse just looks at me strangely and asks, "Why are you on estradiol?"

Now, I expect that maybe these things could come as a surprise to someone who doesn't work in the medical field. I expect more from someone working in an ER (even though this happens to me every single time I've come here, and it always leaves me flabbergasted). I had to answer, in all of the privacy given to me by the sheets which divide beds in an ER, "I'm a trans woman. I'm taking hormones."

The nurse says, "Why, though?"

Seriously? The embarrassment and shame spiral caused by these few simple questions make me want to crawl into a pit and never ever come out. Maybe it would be different if we were talking in a private room, but to have to answer in a place where all of my neighbours could learn a little bit about my (extremely private) medical history and then quietly judge me from their side of the dividing sheets, is mortifying.

I haven't even seen the doctor by this point. It can take some time until the doctor is able to see you, and I'm using this idea as an anchor. Maybe, despite all of these things so far, once I see the actual doctor, the situation will turn around. I hope the doctor has more experience dealing with trans patients than the staff I've seen so far, or if not, maybe just more experience in general, so they would be able to practice empathy and discretion. Maybe some years of working in a hospital will have taught them that, as a patient, I'm looking to be treated like a human who is worthy of respect.

This ends up being a pipe dream. The doctor opens by deadnaming and misgendering me while talking to the nurse who's with him. When I try to correct him, the doctor responds condescendingly with, "Oh! Okay ..." and "Sure ..."

I've made a terrible mistake by choosing to go to the hospital tonight. What makes it infinitely worse is that the doctor has what feels like the loudest voice on the planet. He asks me all of the private and personal questions about being trans—like why I'm on estrogen (really???)—in a voice that you would use when in a noisy place and you're shouting across the room to your friend who's struggling to hear you.

I can't wait for this interview to finish. When it does, he goes back to the nurses' station in the centre of the room surrounded by all of the beds and patients, where he proceeds to recap the interview. In the world's loudest voice. It goes a little something like this:

"HIS NAME IS _____ BUT HE WANTS US TO CALL HIM XEPH. HE WANTS US TO USE FEMALE PRONOUNS. HE'S TAKING SPIRONOLACTONE TO BLOCK TESTOSTERONE, AND ESTRADIOL."

Each sentence feels like I'm being hit with a hammer. In this moment, in my already suicidal state, the doctor has made it a million times worse. I put my coat on, walk out, and end up stumbling around the city for the day and sleeping on the street instead of being in the hospital. Instead of having those whom I trust take care of me, those whose job it is to take care of me, I am now at a brand new low—hopeless, hungry, and cold.

I don't remember how I get home.

The way I was treated in the ER—the misgendering, deadnaming, ignorance, and the lack of discretion I experienced—is incredibly dangerous. When I say it was "my last visit," I mean it. I will not voluntarily return to an ER the next time I'm feeling suicidal. Anything would be a better option than experiencing that level of embarrassment and shame again. Embarrassment and shame, from those who were meant to take care of me.

QUEER AND TRANS HEALTH INNOVATION PROFILE

The Catherine White Holman Wellness Centre (Vancouver, BC)

Fin Gareau, RN and Marria Townsend, MD, Founding Organizers

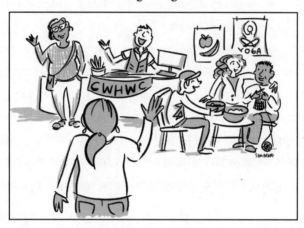

Tell us about the CWHWC and why you're proud of it.

The Catherine White Holman Wellness Centre (CWHWC) is a health and wellness space for trans and gender-diverse people. It's volunteer-run by members of trans, gender-diverse, and queer communities. Trans and gender-diverse people must make up at least 51 percent of the organizers and board members. We work from a set of collective ethics that we developed together.

We offer gender-affirming medical services, counselling, occupational therapy, and sexual health services. We also have yoga, a community kitchen, a nutritionist, an art group, and free legal assistance. We help people with identification changes, access to housing, and pre- and post-surgical care.

We strive to be as low-barrier as we can, and all of our services are free to community members.

We focus on harm reduction and have an informed consent approach to providing gender-affirming care. We offer free injection supplies for people injecting hormones and provide education around self-injection. We work hard to make the waiting room as welcoming as possible, to create a community and social atmosphere.

What changes are you trying to create? What problems are you trying to solve? What does success look like?

We're trying to repair some of the harm that health care providers and the health care system have done to trans people. A lot of trans people are reluctant to access care or don't access care because of these harms. A big part of why we created the centre was to provide a safe space where people would be treated respectfully by care providers who really celebrate who they are, and who want to work with them to get the gender-affirming care they need. We're also trying to lead by example in order to create change in the medical community.

If someone from another place emailed you to say, "I want to do this in my community," and asked for your advice on how to do it, what would you tell them?

The way we evolved was unique. We saw a need, so we got a group of like-minded people together, found a space, and opened our doors. Since then we slowly built a structure around what we were doing. There was work to be done and it couldn't wait. It was obvious that the help was needed. We just had to do it. It felt unethical to stop.

If we were advising somebody else, would we advise them to be more deliberate, thoughtful, to get funding and administrative support in place?

Or would we say, when there's a need, you rise up and you do what needs to be done?

If the CWHWC was gifted $1 million (with no strings attached) by a donor, and your success was completely guaranteed, what would you choose to do?

We'd buy a house so we'd have a space of our own, with a garden and a community kitchen. We'd offer respite and post-op care, and a night shelter so people would have a safe space to come to. Money to pay volunteers would also be good. One day we'll have a house, paid staff, peer programs where people get paid—something sustainable so that we can keep giving back to the community. We'd need more than a million bucks for that!

Is there anything else you'd like to tell us?

Community-building is integral to the CWHWC. Our clinics are more than a place where trans people go for appointments with care providers. People come to us for friendship, support, and conversation. We want all of our clients and volunteers to feel a sense of ownership and belonging. Our volunteers are members of the trans community or closely connected with the community. You can see the relief on new clients' faces when they see themselves reflected in the volunteers—like when an obviously frightened or anxious trans person breathes more easily when they're warmly greeted by our team. We've also built community within our team. We make time to socialize together, to go on annual retreats, and to support each other. There's a depth of caring and commitment to the work that feels like it's only possible because we're family to each other. We hold each other up so that we're better able to hold up our clients.

For more information about the CWHWC, visit cwhwc.com

In my family, if you were an alcoholic, you had a secret.
If you were gay, you were a secret.

WE DON'T HAVE TO NUMB OUT TO BE OUT

Cassia Chambers-Gammill
and Sailor Holladay

The two of us, Cassia and Sailor, have a history of merging drugs and alcohol with family and love and sex and queer identity. We are merging differently here, accounting for where we've been and where we'd like to go. We didn't wake up like this.

Dear Drugs,

You were my first lover. Three years before I ever heated up my first girlfriend's heroin, both of us fourteen, I had you. Paper doses on my tongue, then knife hits burning my lungs. Together we created a baseline of feeling I have forever returned to.

Dear Drugs,

I've used you because I thought I was finding home, because I didn't know where home was, because being home meant feeling not at home, because I remembered home and didn't want to, because I thought I didn't deserve a home. I always crave an elsewhere.

Dear Drugs,

I still think about you, but less. I'm still scared of you, too, which means I'm scared of myself, that I might let you in again, bit by harmless bit, until—

Blackout

I blacked out on my first Valentine's Day with my first girlfriend.

I came out, but I didn't stop blacking out.

I replaced *feeling something* not with *feeling nothing*, but rather with *not feeling*. Erasing myself. Avoidance. Void within A Dance. It's a wonder I survived my survival strategy as long as I did. In a culture that diminishes queer lives, I live and write in and of this body, even while I fear that I have a frightening, unlovable core.

Blackout: drenched in ink without an alphabet. Invisible ink. Can't see my body, ink in my eyes. I can't see you, either. Can't bear any mirrors.

For ten years, choosing to obliterate myself felt more liberated than someone else obliterating me. New Year's Resolution 2005: No More Blackouts. But later, I had a one-night stand with drinking, which led to a one-night stand with blacking out, my hands where they shouldn't be, my insides turned out.

My Family

When my parents, who were addicts, started feeding us kids drugs, there was nowhere to go but up. Drugs and alcohol have tied up my family for so many generations; blame lies in the non-human. Wage labour, incest, war, genocide. That's whose fault it is we have no memory.

In my family, if you were an alcoholic, you had a secret. If you were gay, you *were* a secret. Each supposed flaw with its origin elsewhere; my struggles and desires pathologized. My queerness attributed to mental illness attributed to sexual abuse attributed to alcohol abuse attributed to—what, again? I'm done keeping their secrets. When I give those up, I get something better: my life.

"You're signing up for a very lonely life," my mom said when I came out to her at age fifteen. But my life was already lonely. How much lonelier could it get? The women in my family have always been assigned loneliness, gazing out of curtained windows, their men off at war. A lineage of longing. I never thought I would live to be twenty-one anyway so six more years of misery didn't sound so bad. Especially since I had found that having sex with girls was so much better than with boys and men. With girls, there was a choice to touch.

"When people smoke pot, they take a joint to their lips and inhale," my favorite therapist, Luanna Rodgers, told me. We were in one of our weekly sessions fueled by my hangovers and her compassion. "When *you* smoke pot," she continued, putting her words to twenty years of my feeling, "your whole childhood home goes up in flames."

Gay Family

I regret being too fucked up for so many years to remember the conversations I had with older queers. I regret that getting fucked up was often my priority over having these conversations. I regret that I missed opportunities to listen and gain insight about how to survive and make community amidst hostile environments, live the life you've been told is beyond redemption and repair. I regret I never felt like I was okay enough or that it was enough just to be there with you, the wonder and the treasure of that.

At the end of the night at our favourite gay club, our people, sequined and sloshy, shuffle out, eyes darting everywhere but the door, searching for that someone who—

I've always had to leave San Francisco if I wanted sobriety. Drugs build and tear The City down. The Tech Boom, and before that, Haight-Ashbury, and before that, the Gold Rush.

Our woozy stumbling down Valencia Street just a reiteration of hundreds of lovers before us. Gay bars were at one time a safe space. A place to organize. Now that the Lexington Club has closed, what if we queer women took it as a sign and just. stopped. drinking.

If there's still a queer community, why is it drugs we turn to? Queer folks are three times more likely to abuse drugs and alcohol. That means we should blame ourselves three times less.

Where Is My Body?

My body never belonged to me. Another's pleasure was always more crucial than my own, because of what the absence of their pleasure could mean. Blacking out, I disconnected from my inability to access pleasure in my body. This way, it just didn't have to matter, because I wasn't here anyway.

To have a break from conflict

To be vulnerable

To get on the level

To match my insides to my outsides

To not have to think for a minute

It was that significant to wake up and not be dead. And if someone turned up in my bed? That was even better. Proof that whatever happened last night really happened. For years I didn't know how to flirt, make moves, or have sex without the help of drugs and/or alcohol. A blackout hookup could, the next morning, turn into a year-long relationship. I still haven't figured out how to directly ask someone on a date. Maybe I never will.

Entrypoint

Orientation and disorientation provide a framework for helping me think through my relationship with queerness, drug use, and sobriety.[1] While getting drunk or high is a way of disorienting myself, addiction is a habitual turning of the body and mind in a certain direction, an orientation. Has my addiction been an orientation that has prevented me from claiming other, more desirable orientations? If I'm turning toward drugs, is turning toward queer community even possible? How can I learn to bear the sometimes thrilling, dizzying, and painful disorientations of living as a queer person in a heterosexist structure without relying on substances to cope, connect, commiserate, or celebrate?

Accountability

I quit drinking for good again last November.

I no longer trust someone else telling me who I was last night.

I want to apologize for something I don't remember doing.

I want an apology from someone who doesn't remember doing something to me.

I want to never be in a state of mind again where I could blame my behaviour on a substance.

My apologies are sitting over here in a bucket, first come, first served.

Affirmation (Antidote to Blackout)

We see you.

We see a lot of our people struggling under pretty lights.

We see your resourceful sparkle.

You can act with intention, stay with surprise, and find joy in solitude.

You can feel the hard stuff.

Let it pass through you as you head toward your next iteration.

1 I started thinking along these lines after reading Sarah Ahmed's book *Queer Phenomenology*, which explores the effects of orientations and states of disorientation.

It is important to draw attention to the fact that the social rejection of my trans identity was not only a result of individuals or the hyperpathologization of trans women but also of a society that is not built to support trans youth. Pathology works in such a way that it merely reinforces Western, cissexist paradigms of gender. It does not construct these standards by itself.

DEPATHOLOGIZING TRANS

Eli Erlick

With the recent modifications to the psychiatric model of "transgender" in the *Diagnostic and Statistical Manual of Mental Disorders* (*DSM*), many have questioned the necessity of trans identities being placed among disorders altogether. After years of debate between *DSM*-5 Gender Identity Disorder subworkgroup members, the committee agreed to change "Gender Identity Disorder" to "Gender Dysphoria" as a means to reduce stigma while still retaining the clinical funding and access that comes with a *DSM* diagnosis. While this change is significant, many in the trans community are calling for the complete depathologization of transgender people everywhere. Conceptualizing transness as a mental disorder or pathological condition is not only empirically inaccurate, but also a cause of direct harm to our community.

In 2003, I came out as a queer, transgender girl at eight years old. My mother, a doctor, relied only upon psychiatric and sexological texts to decide if she was going to support me. Unfortunately, transphobic researchers created the prevailing literature on trans and gender nonconforming youth at the time. My mother adhered to the recommended treatments in the book *Gender Identity Disorder and Psychosexual Problems in Children and Adolescents*, written by notorious conversion therapy advocates, Kenneth Zucker and Susan J. Bradley. Their book claimed that if a child's gender identity was not affirmed, they would continue to identify with their sex assigned at birth and live a "normal" (cisgender) life, simply with a greater chance of being queer.

I spent over five years being forced to present in a way that I was not comfortable with, subjecting me to social isolation from the rest of my rural community, intense dysphoria, and assault. I was scared to even acknowledge my gender to myself. I thought I was alone. Being told that I was "wrong" and that "becoming a woman" was impossible prevented me from growing socially. I was not allowed to use the restroom or play on a sports team until high school. The parents of other people my age made sure their children did not interact with me. Had I been allowed to transition, my life would have been greatly improved and I would have been able to have a childhood with friends and support.

While the research found in *Gender Identity Disorder and Psychosexual Problems* has been debunked since the early 2000s, Zucker was the chair of the *DSM-5* Sexual and Gender Identity Disorders Work Group and still wields considerable influence over how trans youth are pathologized. Some cisgender people cling to the notion that they can change their child's identity, just wanting the best life for them. However, this typically causes intense trauma: distress that only started to get notice from mainstream media with the death of Leelah Alcorn in 2014.

It is important to draw attention to the fact that the social rejection of my trans identity was not only a result of individuals or the hyperpathologization of trans women, but also of a society that is not built to support trans youth. Pathology works in such a way that it merely reinforces Western, cissexist paradigms of gender. It does not construct these standards by itself.

When I was finally allowed to medically transition at fifteen, my body became the subject of more pathologization than I was prepared for. I was coerced into feeling as though I would not truly be a trans woman unless I wanted and sought a set of hormonal and surgical interventions that the diagnostic guidelines had predetermined for me. I was very privileged because what I wanted fell roughly into this narrow path. I began hormones when I was fifteen and had gender affirming surgery in the Bay Area when I was seventeen. Both were extremely difficult to obtain. At the time I received hormone therapy, the World Professional Association for Transgender Health Standards of Care dictated that one has to be over the age of sixteen to receive hormonal treatment. Instead of receiving accessible services, I had to go through months of unnecessary therapy and see several doctors to find one who was able to prescribe me the hormones that I needed. I then had to visit several doctors, psychiatrists, and psychologists and fight ageist bias for months to obtain gender affirming surgery before age eighteen.

It was not until after I had surgery and my doctor told me that my entire body looked better that I realized how this medicine can be exploitative of transgender people. I did not feel more "whole" or "complete." Surgery did not have the power to "confirm" my gender. Medical professionals insinuated that my desirability and existence would not be validated until I "fully" transitioned. According to them, I would no longer "feel trapped in the wrong body" (which I never did in the first place). Instead, I simply felt satisfied that I was finally finished with such a large part of my own transition. Perhaps in a society more accepting of women with nonnormative bodies, I would not have needed surgery.

The medicalization of transness that created these conceptualizations will never represent the community as a whole. There is no universal trans experience or biological mechanism. Medicalization will always disadvantage those experiencing intersecting oppressions: denying access to trans people of colour, queer trans people, and trans people with mental illnesses. It also remains empirically flawed. The prevailing medical models of transness try to find neurological foundations for these identities. However, due to neuroplasticity (the brain's ability to change in response to behaviour or environmental factors), identifying with a gender different than the sex assigned at birth can alter the microstructures of the brain in ways that would contrast from a control group of cisgender people.

Many trans people look to these medical models to validate identity. In *Trans Bodies, Trans Selves*, Professor Rachel Levin of Pomona College questions the results of finding a conclusive "trans gene": "If you were to read in tomorrow's newspaper that scientists had found a trans gene, how would you react? ... Would you be less legitimate as a trans or cis person depending on the presence or absence of the gene?" Her critiques of the fixation on a tangible "cause" are justified considering the widespread debate of whether or not we should be putting our resources towards a biological basis of transness instead of transforming society to recognize transgender people's self-determined gender. Along with biological essentialism would come the stigma of "wrongness" and "defect," which would harm the community.

This form of pathologization becomes more complicated due to its support from inside the trans community. While conclusive results would have the potential to decrease social stigma for some, the popularity of finding a "cause" is the result of the medical-industrial complex's grasp on trans legitimacy, something we should decide within our own community. Instead of finding this hypothetical origin, a widespread conceptual model of trans self-determination would be pivotal to transgender liberation. Rather than playing into the oppression of other marginalized groups, the trans community could work in solidarity with them to undo the stigma of determining identity.

Trans people are taking action and pushing back against trans pathologization across the globe. In 2007 Spain passed Law 3/2007, which allowed transgender people to change their names in legal documentation, but only with the costly diagnosis of "gender dysphoria" along with two years of medical treatment. The trans community was outraged. This anger was channeled into organizing and it catapulted Spain into being the international driving force of trans depathological activism with the founding of organizations such as the International Campaign to Stop Trans Pathologization and transnational academic advocacy.

Had these campaigns had more momentum when I was growing up, perhaps my childhood would have been different. I would have not felt ashamed of being trans. I would have been able to easily access the treatment I needed. I would have felt as though my identity was not a "defect," but a gift. The future of trans medicine is bright: more accessible, trans-centred, depathologized practices are coming up around the world. We are looking towards a future in which all trans people can have access to the health care they need, when they need it.

*Illness has been my heavy-handed invitation into transformation, necessitating
close listening, opening to spirit, integrating ancestral trauma while envisioning
new futures, requesting and accepting allyship, and repeated surrender to what is.
These skills translate directly to facilitating healing work.*

THROUGH THE BODY

Fayza Bundalli

I'm twenty-one and my throat is swollen and sore. It's an ordinary moment, feels like any sickness. I don't even remember it clearly. And yet, I'm crossing a threshold into what will begin seven years of bone-deep exhaustion, heavy limbs, loneliness, sharpened intuition, deep listening, losing language.

I am, at this moment, athletic: a runner and a climber. I am a straight-A student and every academic door has opened for me. I am also insecure; later I will connect this to be being brown, to being a child of immigrants, to being queer, and I will learn words like internalized racism and homophobia that will make sense of the way I feel small. I crave belonging, secretly, like a prize I could never win and do not even name.

My family doctor tells me I have mononucleosis. One year later, when I am still sick, she will say I have Chronic Fatigue Syndrome. I have no idea in this moment that I am about to dissolve, that I will reconstitute differently on the other side of this threshold so ordinary I do not even notice myself crossing over.

I'm thirty-one and signing a lease on my own apartment for the first time. I'm living in Oakland, California, and it's my seventh home in just over two years, if we count sublets. Bay Area housing scarcity encourages moves into less-than-perfect roommate situations, and I'm becoming politicized, which decreases my tolerance for bad behaviour. I do not know how to set functional boundaries, but I know how to leave—that skill is in my bones, gifted by great grandmothers and grandfathers and aunties and uncles who've up and left ancestral homes for the sake of safety. I rent my own place for the first time so that I can stop moving; every cell in my body craves rest, and I've dreamed this wood-floored, sunset-facing, claw-foot-bathtub, checker-tile-backsplash studio apartment into life.

Two months later, I am in bed for four days. Each day I feel worse. By the end of the week I am shaking and unsteady. I cannot breathe, cannot think when I am exposed to chemicals, and chemicals are everywhere: the pilot light on the stove, white-board markers at work, cleaners and fragrances in most public places, on most people. I am terrified and feel like I have no skin. I ask my landlord if any work was done to the apartment before I moved in, and learn that the kitchen floor was replaced, new laminate and glue off-gassing into the tiny apartment. I also learn that my mattress, like most new mattresses, was saturated with fire retardant including formaldehyde.

I am at another beginning: this time the transition is dramatic, and I am scared. Having dissolved completely through illness once before, I know what the losses can be. I do not take for granted the pleasures of being body to body in friendships, of having a simpler relationship to work, of being able to predict my energy and follow through on commitments. I am not ready, I am not willing.

My body does not ask if I am ready, willing. I am curled into a ball on the wood floor, arms hugging my knees, holding myself together from the outside. I have washed my hands with scented soap in a rash attempt to show myself that I am okay, and now my limbs tremor and ache, my lungs heavy and reluctant to take in breath, my brain plunged into fog and confusion. I am frozen with fear, in some way unreachable as my body once again crosses over a threshold beyond which there is no intact return.

I'm twenty-one, and withdraw from classes, move in with my parents. I lie in bed. I muster up the energy to shower and return to rest. I muster up the energy to eat, and return to rest. My brain is full of sensation, lost to thought, my legs are full of ache. I have not completed the trajectory, not accomplished the successes that I thought made me good. Instead I am listening closely to my body; what else is there to do? Yes, no, how much. I become well enough to walk outside, and do so slowly, rest on every bench, carry sunglasses and a book, nap everywhere.

Over time almost every friend drops away, and I let them go; even phone calls are most often too much for my capacity. I grow a loneliness that will be difficult to shake, even years later, even when I hear daily from partner, from family, from friends how dearly I am loved.

My family doctor tells me Chronic Fatigue Syndrome is a mystery and she has nothing to offer beyond a diagnosis. The first time I am well enough to walk to the ocean near my parents' house, I see a poster advertising the work of a medical intuitive. I call her, and she becomes my first mentor in this strange landscape through which I have no map. She sees inside my body, talks to spirit guides; she tells me about intergenerational trauma, how it is carried in my body, how I have directed my anger inwards and the seams are blowing open. I learn about the impacts of displacement, how racism over generations has left my body vulnerable. This healer has also been sick and has learned her skills through her own body; she speaks to me, and knows, as only one who has gone before can.

Illness sensitizes my body to spirit; it is a gateway through which some of us walk between worlds. When I am crashed out, when every muscle of my back contacts the mattress and I do not have the strength or stamina to sit up, some dial on my connection to and communication with spirit turns up. I have vivid dreams, see things that do not have physical form, and have sudden knowings. I also have a visceral sense of well-being that cannot be shaken by my physical state of illness.

One such night, it is suddenly necessary to tell my first queer crush and closest friend that I love her, I will not heal unless I do; in the morning, more rested, I decide this is irrational, and besides, I have a boyfriend. When I gather the courage two years later and too late to win her, I learn that acknowledging queer desire is needed at the centre of my healing. On another such afternoon, my older cousin who has died some years earlier keeps me company as I heat my lunch. He was my steady teammate through childhood summers of playing outside. That afternoon, I am weak with fatigue and he's there, steady.

I am thirty-one and move back to Vancouver, land in my parents' home once more. I move slowly, listen to trees, to birds, to the ocean. I acclimatize to living with Multiple Chemical Sensitivity (MCS) in the ways that I can, meaning I am frequently sick and re-learning my body. The first time in a long while that I make plans to see a film, I am flushed with shame telling a new friend I will need to wear a mask. He lights up and says, "I'll wear a mask too."

I mix a herbal tincture with water three times a day, drink the bitter that shakes out my limbs and contorts my face. The herbalist I see had MCS as a child and knows how to treat it. His tinctures coax my system down from hairline reactivity, flush toxins from my organs, teach my cells to rebuild safety. I am again deeply impacted by a healer who has been sick, who has learned through his own body and makes an informed offering. This is the type of healer I am learning to be.

I am thirty-five and have opened a somatic therapy practice. My work grounds in my body, connection with spirit, and the teachings of my mentors. Somatics rebuilds connection to the body and sensation as avenues of knowing and healing; it's life-affirming towards the all-of-it that life is. Healing through the body is not a neutral choice: the felt sensation of fatigue lays me flat, chemical toxicity in my tissues curls me up. Increasing connection to my body requires feeling into the full range of what's there.

Illness has been my heavy-handed invitation into transformation, necessitating close listening, opening to spirit, integrating ancestral trauma while envisioning new futures, requesting and accepting allyship, and repeated surrender to what is. These skills translate directly to facilitating healing work. Many of us who live or have lived with illness make critical contributions to collective healing. Through illness I have decomposed and regrown different, to know, finally, that a life that includes chronic illness is as deeply necessary as every other, as worthy of belonging, as important to our collective freedoms.

My healing is not my own, because health and healing occur beyond just that
which is held within a single body.

HEALING EXCHANGES

the necessity of beloved community for queer survivors of colour

Ariel Estrella

My healing is not my own. It can't be, not as a queer Latinx survivor of violence. It can't be, not when it was trauma that first introduced my body to how much my health and survival rely on others' presence in my life. I burned the word "interdependence" under my skin when my lethargic depression fed my relative Emmanuel's violent depression in a toxic loop of aching familiarity. I realized collectivity at the sight of a staircase where I pressed my feet against a banister to prevent me from being tossed down the steps. I drew out my intersectionality witnessing family members jumped by their fathers for seeming too much like a *maricón*.

When I began healing, I experienced the desperate need for a more comprehensive inclusion of beloved community. I was still technically surviving then, keeping the abuse secret because I didn't want to start any trouble. Following a week-long stay in an in-patient ward after I told an emergency room nurse I was suicidal, my high school told me I was required to see a psychiatrist for my continued enrolment. It was an illegal mandate, but my family and I had no way to know otherwise.

229

I didn't like Dr. Weiss. She was a white woman with a flighty body tucked into edges beneath the same black top and gray tweed pants she wore every week. And every week, she frustrated me with how much I needed her to understand me. I wasted time contextualizing my queerness, my family, and myself; I wanted her to just understand them intrinsically. Even after my explanations, she would push aside topics I considered important, such as my budding queer identity, because we were meant to prioritize my abuse recovery. I saw and still see my identities and experiences as tightly woven together, in ways I would have been happy to explore, but she compartmentalized my life as she saw fit. I felt empty. The meds made me productive to a point, but the detachment I felt between my actions and my emotions unnerved me. Our relationship reflected that detachment.

It was not just that she was white, straight, and cisgender. What set her apart from other white, straight, cisgender medical providers I've had is that she was cold. She was distant in a way I never experienced within any of my Latinx and/or queer communities, up to and including Emmanuel's treatment of me. Dr. Weiss maintained a strictly clinical distance, following the tradition of white western practices. As a Latinx queer from New York, I measured care in terms of emotional reciprocity. Because for beloved communities like ours—where you might not speak the dominant language, or where you might gesture to queerness for safety, but never implicate yourself fully within it—nonverbal cues are a vital means of communication. You drop your bland subway face in the presence of your compadres, your cousins and your "cousins," and chosen fam (who in my case included my bio fam). You pass everywhere else as less than your full emotional self, as needed for survival. What she was giving me did not provide the adequate comfort required for deeper healing in my cultural context for care.

I once stayed silent for forty-three minutes of a forty-five-minute session in retaliation. The previous session I had noticed that she spoke only after I addressed her and I wanted to see how far her conversational tactic would go. The imposed silence was an unkind test of her patience, but that mattered little to me then. My compassion waned in a jealousy for the power she held over our conversations.

So I stared, and I stared at her clock, and I stared at her ugly paintings, and I stared at the murky sky through the window behind her, and I waited for her to break.

I don't remember what she said at the forty-four-minute mark, but I know that any pride over my victory soured quickly with the realization that I would be back for more the following week. I left the office that day with a choking slick of saliva building up at the back of my throat. I walked away burning for her to be what I needed her to be: someone like me.

While I couldn't believe it sitting in her office, I knew that aspects of her methodology appealed to some people. I also knew that other providers would have different techniques, but I did not think to seek help elsewhere. I was raised to be deeply suspicious of mental health services, in part because of the relative inaccessibility of appropriate mental health education and services for people of colour. Shrinks were for white people, I was told, and pills were for crazy white people who couldn't take care of themselves. Shame spiked into the mere fact that I needed help; to be picky about the person I wanted to see was just another failure on top of everything else.

I kept going until I couldn't. I eventually got a letter in the mail that Dr. Weiss cancelled all of our future appointments.

The scope of the treatment Dr. Weiss offered was limited. She had set up strict boundaries to my recovery that didn't consider the fluidity of my intersectional life or my needs as a queer Latinx. I needed to talk about the trauma of witnessing queerphobia and knowing there would be further violence if word got out about my queerness. I needed to address the fear that my trans identity came from a desire to be like the men in my family, backed by the hope a more masculine persona could offer me protection within a *maschista* paradigm. I needed to be reassured that I was not a traitor for speaking out about abuse outside the family. I needed to heal, an act of transformation that values holistic wellness of heart, soul, and the beloved communities necessary to support reflection.

Frustrated by the failure with Dr. Weiss, I continued without treatment of any explicit kind for years, stumbling through with the constant pressure of depression and anxiety, risking any hard-earned gains. Halfway through college and a thousand miles away from my family, though, I couldn't continue on as I was. Ignoring the issue wasn't helping. So I sought therapy with practitioners more suited to me, but even with the stabilization offered to me by my medical providers, counsellors, and medication, I wanted deeper care.

I didn't have to look far. I found community with other queer Latinx survivors of violence, with whom I did my most targeted healing. We found each other by accident and through trust built over time, and my participation in a collective for Latin American women and non-binary folk of the diaspora brought me intimately close to the conversations I desperately needed to take part in. There, I found myself beloved to those who I loved dearly. There, I found people to call my soul hermanx, my siblings, our solidarities forged through our survivorhood and profound ability to love.

Through our shared histories, through feeling resonances of my pain in theirs, through our vulnerability and strength, through mentorship, I steadied myself.

One mentor, Gabe, gave me the support I only dreamed of when I first started thinking through my need for beloved community. We ate together every now and again, knowing that for both of us Latinx folx, sharing food was an intimate kindness. Over a plate of Afghani in mid-February, we talked around our full mouths, our conversation easy yet urgent with an intensity I missed from New York City life. We swayed from my difficulties with white queer activism on campus to the topic of depression. He stopped spearing his salad to tell me about his experience with the depths depression takes us to as queer Latinx survivors and how we cling to survival. He told me about time he spent institutionalized for depression, how it sucks, but that it's an option that no one should feel ashamed of needing.

He was the first Latinx I knew other than myself who had experienced in-patient treatment. For years I had hidden the fact that I had been institutionalized, guarding the secret *con vergüenza*. I bawled loudly in the near-empty cafe just knowing I was not alone. It wasn't just that he lived through it, but that he lived and healed. He still dealt with PTSD episodes from time to time. He still remembered his traumas with pain. And he was still around. For someone who, for nearly a decade, didn't imagine making it through the day, I never imagined myself with a future.

His survival was my own. Within him, within his joy and pain, success and family and breath, I saw myself.

By sharing my experience with him, Gabe and I built the healing reciprocation that was so missing from the clinical treatment practices that isolated me. Our conversation was an instance of a beloved community between two people. Our friendship expands that bond as we use our conversations to inspire others.

Years later, and my healing is still not my own. It can't be, not when I flinch as a colleague approaches my desk from behind and lays a hand on my shoulder to catch my attention. My body jolts upwards, possessed by a memory pulling from the base of my skull. I feel the years-old ache of Emmanuel's hand around my ponytail, yanking me backwards as I stumbled towards *mi mamá*'s apartment for help. My healing is trigger-split between the presence of my teenaged trauma, the effect of people past and present, and the mental disembodiment that accompanies peaks in my anxiety.

My healing is not my own, not fully, because I'm not really sure how I got here. Years of depression and PTSD and anxiety shredded my information retention; save for my tactile and emotional memory, my recall is utterly shot. But with so few facts to ground me, I sense more than I know myself. I am a fissure of repeated narratives I tell and have other people tell me. My healing, then, is not really my own because even if I could, I wouldn't want to jealously hold myself to a singular vision of personhood as I move ever forward.

My healing is not my own.

It can't be because I am a multiplicity: by circumstance of trauma, by the interactions I have with the world around me, and by necessity of the narratives that construct who I am. I'm more than just myself, a philosophy I learned early as I bore my family's every sacrifice and success and pride. Queerness, latinidad, queer latinidad, and the solidarities I engage in as a person of colour extend this vision of collectivity to all parts of my life. Through my identities and explorations of self, I not only found support and love and tenderness, but peers, friends, mentors, and even strangers with understanding smiles. With them we found one another with such care, and a tenderness I came to understand as beloved community. Even before I realized I was healing, even before I opened up about my traumas, they gave me life.

My healing is not my own, because health and healing occur beyond just that which is held within a single body. For me, healing as a survivor is not (only) for the purpose of stabilizing my ability to handle the day-to-day, it is also a constant action; it is a verb seeking renegotiations of self as the contexts change over time. Beloved community acts as both a witness to and participant in this process through healing exchanges of intimacy shared along atoms, esters, echoes of our ancestors, embraces after hours-long conversations, *bruja* superstitions, and the accidental brush of a fellow strap-hanger during a morning commute.

The refusal to center individuality through healing after trauma may be frightening because to do so is simultaneously difficult, time consuming, painful, and at times a dangerous act of resistance. For survivors, there's only so much we can give. There is only so much interaction we can tolerate. There is only so much we can love and cherish when our bodies ache and tear for an instant cure.

For truly sustainable living, however, we must question any long-term methods of healing that isolate the survivor. These methods may contribute to an individualism that is (riffing off bell hooks) ableist colonial cissexist heterocentric white supremacist capitalist patriarchal and all ways otherwise oppressive. Limiting the view of healing after trauma upholds the exact individualism that isolates survivors of multiply marginalized communities from one another and the resources we desperately need.

Any one person is more than just themself, so an individual's health must be understood alongside one's beloved community. Forming healing communities with fellow queer Latinx survivors like Gabe saved my life. And yes, it can be difficult at times. With all of us similarly traumatized and healing, we trigger one another. We sometimes can't afford the energy or time to support each other. The trial of collective healing after individualized violence can be taxing, but it's usually outweighed by the beloved potential of finding support with one another. Our individual healing becomes the healing of a community, balanced between the love bound through our intersections.

Anti-racism and anti-abuse activism is vital to ill-health prevention for queer and trans people of colour. Understanding how to better care for our multiply marginalized survivors will bring us all up together, instead of supporting just one axis of identity in our activism. By focusing on beloved communities, I can heal. I still have PTSD and I am (and expect to always be) anxious, but now I stand in solidarity with beloveds who hold me accountable to my emotional, spiritual, and community health.

My healing is not my own, because I am not alone.

I am the midnight conversations over Facebook, and the jokes over a pot of black beans, and the days we never thought we would have.

I am dust and dirt and grime and Goya.

I am a community, healed and healing, beloved and forever loving.

It was liberating to work someplace queer and trans positive, where I could confidently refer members of communities I was a part of. I was also engaging in subconscious integration of my own trauma as a direct result of working in a clinic designed to be as safe as possible for trauma survivors. Trauma-informed clinics recognize the widespread impact of trauma, actively resist re-traumatizing people, and try to restore a sense of safety.

NOT A LIABILITY
On Trauma-Informed Care and Community Acupuncture
Lisa Baird

I owe my livelihood to the work of the Black Panthers and the Young Lords. When I sat down to write about trauma-informed care and my work in community acupuncture, I knew I had to share some of the neglected origin story of community acupuncture in North America. It wasn't until I was immersed in the writing of it that I realized that community acupuncture as trauma-informed care is intimately tied to the historical efforts of the Panthers and the Lords to heal trauma at a community level. The roots of the community acupuncture movement are more than fascinating social history.

Acupuncture is one of the oldest, simplest, and safest forms of health care in the world. It has traditionally been practiced in group settings, with people receiving as much treatment as needed. In China, acupuncture is an established component of the health care system, and acupuncture treatment costs the equivalent of two or three dollars. Unfortunately, in North America today, most acupuncture schools train students to treat one patient per hour, with practitioners charging anywhere from $50-

$150 per session, such that regular treatment is out of the question for most people. The community acupuncture (CA) movement is working to change this. Community acupuncturists (referred to as "acupunks") charge patients on a sliding scale, somewhere between $15 and $40 per treatment. Patients decide for themselves what they can afford, no questions asked.

The CA movement has roots in the social struggles of the 1960s and '70s, specifically the Black Panther Party and Young Lords movements. The Black Panther Party was a revolutionary Black socialist organization fighting for employment and housing for Black people, challenging police brutality, and providing "survival programs" such as free food and medical care, clothing distribution, lessons in self-defence and first aid, and an emergency-response ambulance program. The Young Lords were an anti-racist, anti-imperialist community organization striving for Puerto Rican self-determination, often focusing on health care.

Several delegations of Panthers studied acupuncture in China. Upon their return, free medical care for the Black community became an increasing focus of Panther activity. In 1970, the Lords and the Panthers took over Lincoln Hospital—known by the community as the "butcher shop of the South Bronx"[1]—in response to the denial of adequate medical care for their communities. For a brief period in the 1970s, members of the Lords and the Panthers worked alongside socially conscious doctors and health care workers at the Lincoln Hospital.

The now-famous Lincoln Detox (established as a direct result of work by the Lords and the Panthers) offered group acupuncture treatments to support withdrawal from drugs. In the early days, the hugely successful Lincoln Detox program included political education alongside group acupuncture

1 Vicente "Panama" Alba, interview with Molly Porzig, "Lincoln Detox Center: The People's Drug Program," The Abolitionist (blog), March 15, 2013. https://abolitionistpaper.wordpress.com/2013/03/15/lincoln-detox-center-the-peoples-drug-program.

treatments. Participants learned about the role of governmental institutions such as the CIA in drug trafficking in poor and racialized neighbourhoods, and the relationship of prohibition to the maintenance of social control. Lincoln Detox was targeted by the FBI under COINTELPRO, and over 200 members of the New York Police Department (including SWAT teams) used excessive force to close it down in 1979.

Lincoln Detox became the model for many other acupuncture detoxification (AcuDetox) centers in public health clinics worldwide. In 1985, Dr. Michael Smith and others founded the National Acupuncture Detox Association (NADA) to provide an outside mechanism for certifying practitioners in the NADA acupuncture protocol. This has allowed AcuDetox to flourish, so that it is currently used by approximately one thousand addiction treatment programs in North America and abroad. Political consciousness raising, however, is not currently a component of AcuDetox treatment.

The roles of the Lords and the Panthers in the spread of acupuncture in North America are often dismissed or omitted. It was the AcuDetox model that inspired the CA model as practiced today. As community acupuncturists, we owe our livelihoods to the Black Panthers and the Young Lords.

I didn't learn any of this history in college.

Acupuncture school was challenging for me. I was hit hard by the pervasive cultures of sexism and homophobia at both colleges I attended. My five years studying Traditional Chinese Medicine (TCM) included an unapologetically homophobic anatomy and physiology professor and sexual harassment from more than one male student.

I loved learning about TCM, however, and was one of the busiest practitioners in the student clinic. My patients were almost all members of queer and/or trans communities and I treated a range of symptoms related to trauma (depression, anxiety, body pain, insomnia). I was happy to be busy—but I was also under-supported. Confidentiality agreements meant that I couldn't speak to friends about my clinical work. Peer support from other students or supportive clinical supervision from my teachers were unattractive options—I didn't want to confirm anyone's suspicions that queer and trans people are basically unwell. There was no one I could talk to about my suicidal patients, my self-harming patients, or my patients with night terrors. I carried that alone.

There was no discussion at acupuncture school of structural violence, of the impacts of normalized trauma, of who becomes chronically ill and why. We were encouraged to give importance to diet and lifestyle counselling ("You can't help someone who won't help themselves") with no comment on how living with the steady threat of transphobic violence, for example, might contribute to a scorching case of gastric reflux and how that patient might then actually be harmed, not helped, by a potentially shaming lecture from a practitioner on avoiding coffee and other acid-forming foods. There was a deep and unspoken disconnect between what happened in the classroom and the reality of my work in the student clinic.

I couldn't articulate back then that marginalized folk are disproportionately affected by trauma, that trauma has impacts on health, that I didn't want to position myself as an expert on anyone else's life, that I needed to meet my patients where they were at, that holistic medicine should account for all aspects of people's lives.

As a queer-identified young woman with a trauma history, I was trying to offer trauma-informed care and harm reduction to highly traumatized members of communities of which I was a part, in an educational setting which was re-traumatizing to me on a daily basis.

I graduated from acupuncture school with no idea of how to make a living doing acupuncture. I knew that charging my patients upwards of $50 per treatment would not work for me, ethically or practically. The people

I wanted to treat—friends and family—would not be able to afford those rates. Fortunately, when I was ready to start practicing, I discovered Poke Community Acupuncture in my Vancouver neighbourhood and the owner gave me a job. Patients were charged on a sliding scale of $20-$40 per treatment and treated in recliners in a large quiet room together.

My first months working at Poke involved extensive retraining as I learned how to give effective distal style acupuncture treatments in a group setting (using points below the knees and elbows, and on the head) and, just as importantly, spent hours reading posts on the Community Acupuncture Network (which has since evolved into an international cooperative, the People's Organization of Community Acupuncture, or POCA). The online conversations gave me a broader context and deeper meaning for my work. I was treating hundreds of people and I was also a part of an international movement, connected through my work to hundreds of other practitioners and thousands of patients.

It was liberating to work someplace queer and trans positive, where I could confidently refer members of communities I was a part of. I was also engaging in subconscious integration of my own trauma as a direct result of working in a clinic designed to be as safe as possible for trauma survivors. Trauma-informed clinics recognize the widespread impact of trauma, actively resist re-traumatizing people, and try to restore a sense of safety. Community acupuncture clinics are designed to be trauma-informed.

In a CA clinic, everything from intake to treatment happens out in the open. Patients are very rarely alone with a practitioner. CA clinics are predictable; patients learn what to expect by observing what is happening around them. People who are nervous about acupuncture can come for treatment with friends and family, which creates additional social safety. The CA model emphasizes choice: patients choose what they can afford to pay on the sliding scale, which chair they sit in, whether they want to recline or sit upright, and how long they stay. Given the diversity of treatment strategies available, treatment can easily be adapted for a patient's comfort. If someone doesn't want to remove their socks or roll up their trouser legs, for example, we simply choose different points on the body. There is never any need to push a patient to expose any part of their body.

I quickly learned that with regular, frequent treatment, acupuncture alone can often produce remarkable results. The CA model discourages dietary and lifestyle advice. The only recommendation we gave our patients at Poke was when to come back for more treatment.

Previous to my work in CA, almost all of my patients had been cisgendered women or trans folk. At Poke I was treating people of all genders, including many cisgendered men, which was surprisingly healing for me. I had a deep distrust of cisgendered men throughout my twenties. Being subtly alarmed by cis males is an exhausting way to spend a decade; I don't recommend it. I still recall with utter tenderness the first cis man I befriended, and the second, and the third. It was a really big deal. Through my work in CA, I was having regular, straightforward, and meaningful interactions with cis men who weren't trying to hurt me. I was very rarely alone with them, and they were coming to me for help—that is, with some degree of vulnerability—in a setting where it was safe for me to care about them. Cis men as regular folk with frailties and struggles and simple human gratitude for pain relief: this is a part of what I was learning and experiencing. It was no longer a big deal. It became normal. It burned new neural pathways in my survivor's brain.

People with trauma histories often end up being hyper-vigilant and very aware of others' moods and feelings. This is a useful quality for surviving unpredictable and violent situations, but again, it is exhausting to be on high-alert in every situation and can make one-on-one caregiving interactions exceptionally draining.

In the group treatment room, however, even the most upset or anxious patients are "held" by the group and generally nap with their needles alongside everyone else. My job is to give patients treatment, then be aware of when they need another blanket, when a needle has to be adjusted, or when it is time to end the treatment. The treatment room is space for my heightened awareness without the accompanying alarm. I get to learn a way of being open-hearted and present with others' pain and unmet needs without feeling responsible for fixing them or fearing the consequences of not fixing them. What I had previously named my over-sensitivity does not hurt me in this setting; it's actually one of the reasons I'm good at my job.

Many of us who were abused as children have been conditioned to care for our abusers. This easily translates to codependent patterns as adults: a disproportionate sense of responsibility for others. The phenomenon of community *qi*—of the synchronization of acupuncture patients into a state of harmony and deep relaxation while the needles do their work—has interrupted those patterns in me. Being able to set needles for someone in absolute crisis and then turn to the next person, trusting that everyone will be held safely enough by the room, continues to be a powerful contradiction to my storyline of needing to take care of everyone myself.

In my first six months at Poke, I experienced a traumatic event and learned firsthand the effectiveness of acupuncture as an intervention for the impacts of trauma. The other acupuncturists at Poke gave me daily acupuncture for over a week. I cried, then slept, before or after my shifts, often alongside my regular patients, every day.

One of the deepest wounds I have carried as someone with a trauma history has been the requirement that I smile through pain, that I always appear as though I've got it together, that I'm just fine, thank you. Bringing my entire self to work has gone a long way towards mending the internal splits caused by years of forced smiles.

Healing from trauma is cyclical, nonlinear, and unpredictable. There are good days, bad days, and strange numb days. There are days that start out with early morning nightmares, with struggling to get to clinic with enough time to sweep the treatment room (too tired to do it the night before), that become one of the best days I've ever had, as my regular patients fill the treatment room with their pain, their resilience, their rest. There are days of thought-free integration of my own wounding as I engage with the wounds of others. There are exchanges with traumatized patients who have never had acupuncture before, who are possibly wary of another violation, and the silent recognition between survivors when I let them know that I'll stop if they say the word, as I ask permission to touch their wrist. There's the moment of release as they realise they're safer than they thought, that this might actually be okay.

POCA's latest project is POCATech, an affordable acupuncture school for community acupuncturists.[2] The curriculum includes a significant focus on the history of acupuncture in North America and on trauma-informed care. Trauma-informed care workshops have become a regular part of CA gatherings (POCAFests). A growing number of us are not only recognizing that trauma is as widespread among practitioners as it is among patients, but also articulating our experiences as competent community acupuncturists who are still impacted by our trauma histories and deeply affected by our work.

A history of trauma can leave us with a lingering sense of shame around being broken. Health care providers with trauma histories are under enormous pressure to be completely healed and maintain composure. This pressure to be "whole" persists despite the fact that those of us who have had

2 POCATech students learn Liberation Acupuncture, "a conceptual framework for acupuncture that affirms that individual health and disease do not exist, and cannot be understood or addressed, apart from social conditions—particularly injustice, inequality, and the pervasive influence of traumatic stress."

to navigate re-traumatizing health care systems are sometimes best able to offer care that is trauma-informed. A trauma history is *not* a liability for those of us working in health care.

I struggle to express what it has meant for me to have respected colleagues who are also dear friends, who are also trauma survivors. Having allies who can respond to my text saying "Got triggered in clinic last night, still kinda shaky this morning, have had three drop-ins today, all in crisis" with "Oh, hon. Hang in there, I love you." They stitch me back together when I'm falling apart, affirm that wholeness is not a requirement, healing is not a destination, and that we don't do this alone.

I listen to their histories, their frustrations and their life stories, writing none of it down. I ask what their names are, and assure them that I mean their own names, not the ones that Authority demands for paperwork. I open my eyes and heart as wide as I can, and I listen.

LISTEN

Sossity Chiricuzio

It's 1976, and I'm face down on the big chrome table, trying to hold still despite the row of tiny buttons on my favorite dress pressing up into my stomach and chest, my right eye swollen shut and purple. My mom is whispering forcefully, and the X-ray tech is brusque, and it's all related to how a six-year-old kid can end up looking like this. The question of why I was jumping off the back of a parked car is reasonable, but the grown-up they should be asking isn't here. He never is, except right before I'm hurt.

"Jump," he says, "I'll catch you," and he does the first few times, and I keep jumping, even though being caught by him is the opposite of safety. The third time he steps forward and slips on some loose gravel, and I'm already airborne. Below me is his fearful face, and that's almost worth the crash into the brick wall that follows, and the drop to the gravel, and the scraping slide that has brought me here, balanced on my tiny buttons.

This is actually the least scary thing he does to me, and the only one the doctors ever check. The only one my mother knows about. The only one that heals quickly.

In comparison with the almost four decades that follow, he is a blip. Participating in our extended community just enough to seem known, he has me in his hands maybe a half dozen hours all told, and yet. It's still his hands, forcing me into positions and invading my body, that give teeth and snarls to my dreams. It's his voice, silencing mine, that I have to overcome again and again to have conversations about what I need and what I want. He cast himself as Authority over my body, and I believe him for far too long.

Another twelve years, more invaders and their silencing voices, and I am pliant, empty, and exhausted. The last man I'm with breaks the condom, turns out to be a carrier of HPV, is barely sorry. A sympathetic nurse makes him watch the biopsy, my cervix projected onto the screen a foot across and bleeding until he loses all colour, but I'm the one with scars. On the second visit the doctor gives me a big orange Tylenol, mumbles something about being more careful next time, and aims the laser between my legs. I am splayed, helpless until it's done.

The same nurse finally explains that every three months I will have to get a full exam to make sure the precancerous cells were all burned away. The frustration and shame of that is a low flame compared to the torture of telling the lesbian couple that had finally turned me out after months of chasing them and answers about myself. I didn't know about the HPV before we had our fling, and the concept of "No glove, no love" hadn't reached the nowhere desert town we lived in. No symptoms, just a routine yearly like my mother has drummed into me, and then the gut-punch feeling of bringing disease into that tender circle we'd made.

Every trip to the clinic brings another round of invasive questions and disclosure and defense and education with Authority. Then the silence, while the layer of latex between us takes the shape of me, their hand, feeling for flaws. I leave a detailed reading list of books and articles about sexuality and gender and body image. I wait for the phone call, start breathing again once it comes. I never once have an appointment without having to defend my sexuality or sexual choices. I never again have sex without protection, even in love, even in a hurry, unless I'm fluid bound with that person.

In that same year I get the flu, and my bones catch fire. I drag myself to the community clinic, wait two hours for the dead-eyed doctor to tell me what's wrong. The ground glass in my joints makes it clear this is not just the flu. "Arthritis," he says, "just have to live with it." I'm stunned into silence, even as I fill up with rage. Barely eighteen, surprised to still be alive. So many years spent thinking I would stumble into dying, numb almost to the point of it. Ready to finally enjoy life, my body, and then this. Like my bones are older than me. Like a punishment, though I don't believe in that, or rather in any deity who would take the time to punish one mote of dust for bending left.

I can't fathom the diagnosis, and can't escape it. I'm scraping by since I came out, losing some family and many friends, hating the skin I'm in, and now the bones as well. Lonesome baby dyke, my only real connection the closeted late night DJ at the radio station. She keeps me company for the first part of my graveyard shifts as I dispatch cabs with decreasing frequency, sends me a bootleg cassette of the first album by Melissa Etheridge. The value of that tiny gesture spotlights my desperation, even for me. I'm passing community college but completely uninspired. I sometimes think about dying, but hold on with aching fingers. Stubborn.

The women in my family have long served as the gatekeepers of the medical field. The voice of reason and soothing, the glue that keeps the mechanics humming. Billing, records, nurses' station, ward clerk, lab tech, stand-in mother, collective memory bank, go-to plan that is almost never credited. Knowing everything but denied Authority, they keep people from falling through the cracks. Keep the doors open and the lights on. Keep going to work even past the joy of it, knowing they make a difference. Knowing that it costs them, and also, that the work is vital. Sacred, even, beyond the bureaucracy and draining details.

I want more. Want to not be caught up in everybody's need for everything right now, watching my weekend dribble away into catching up on sleep and laundry. I am full of hunger, my belly tight with it, my bones a hot drumming under the skin of my hands. I wonder if it's my fault, for those mirrors and walls I beat my thwarted teenage fists against when no one would listen. Right there, where the centre knuckle rises higher—is that loathing or inflammation? That stab of hot steel through the centre of my hand—the clench of rage or disease? I can't escape my body, but I at least have to get out of this tiny town.

My one constant is my mother, who is also my best friend, and ready for more in her life. We take the leap together. Register for the big city university, start gulping down knowledge and spreading roots, building our overlapping lives. Full of joy even when the glow begins to wear thin after months of ramen. We're not just filling in the blanks, we're listening to stories and learning truths Authority has tried to erase. The black and brown and red and yellow voices. The female and young and disabled voices. The outlaws and outcasts. Scrubbing away at the whitewashing. So heady, pushing back against the status quo. Breathing it in like the steam of cold water meeting red coals. Breathing out No.

I join the Gay and Lesbian Alliance and start fighting for inclusion of bisexuals; join ACT UP and get involved in the fight for a cure; join Queer Nation and fight for sexual freedom and education; join the Lesbian Avengers and fight for safe streets at night. I argue with the library about their lack of texts on queer theory, with my professors about the types of feminism they teach, with other dykes about kink and femininity, with my old friends about politics and sexuality. I argue with anyone who tries to fit me into one neatly labeled box. It's not just for the sake of arguing; I am on a mission of change. For myself, and how I move through the world.

Eventually Authority declares my cervix safe, and I begin to relax. The fire in my bones subsides deep into my joints, flaring only at extreme cold or exertion. I revel in my strength and share it easily, so when I do limp or falter it shocks people. I hate it, hide it, the only secret left in the closet. Hard enough to get jobs that require heavy lifting. Hard enough to walk through the world with muscles and skirts, or to get queers to hand over the power tools without questioning my gender. Wider discussions about ability are rare, and I often push too far or go without, just to avoid having to disclose or ask for help. I leave college knowing there is no place for my voice there yet. Back to working with my hands, whetting my mind against poetry and politics.

When the pain does flare up, I try every remedy suggested. I find that Western medicine leaves me sick to my stomach, and still in pain. What does help is a folk remedy widely used but rarely discussed: Marijuana. Taking the edge off enough to keep walking, or working, it is both cheaper and easier to find. The research about this at the time is limited, but I learn how to ease my pain. Topical and edible options, the science of THC vs CBD,[1] and their receptors in our brains. I have to dig for information on this potent little plant but the reward is immediate, especially when used in conjunction with alternative bodywork.

I've always enjoyed massage, but as I befriend more massage therapists, I begin to discover the power of medical massage. How their knowledge and manipulation of muscles and joints and tendons can help keep my body in motion and my pain levels down. In turn, they introduce me to folks who do acupuncture, a practice that seems magical in the use of needles so slender they rarely even draw blood. Pressure points and chi, hold and slide and release, healing hands on my body, giving it back to me. I trade any skill I have for the benefits they can offer, and with every session I feel my body become more solid, more mine.

I spend the next several decades doing every kind of labour that will pay the bills: cooking and serving food, cleaning houses and offices, shelving

---

1 THC (tetrahydrocannabinol) is the psychoactive ingredient in cannabis. CBD (cannabinoid) is the non-psychotropic ingredient that's shown to have anti-inflammatory and muscle-relaxing properties.

library books, yard work, slinging red clay into heavy molds, endless hours of data entry and coding, and unloading and selling furniture. That last job puts the final wear and tear on my shoulders, eventually sending me into a tailspin of jagged pain spikes and the inability to lift more than five pounds at a time. Feeling broken and scared, I force myself to go to the chiropractor, hoping she can quickly put something back into place so I can get on with my life. As if anything is ever that simple.

Tendons have shifted out of place, joints are tired and twisted, and even my nerves are pinched. Both arms, out of commission indefinitely. I have some trade banked with the chiropractor from years ago, that plus her sympathy results in an offer to treat me for a month. Four times a week I spend the day shuttling back and forth on a bus, trying not to cry from pain and frustration. Unable to clean my house, carry groceries, pull my lover into an embrace. They use ultrasound, drop tables, activators, and traction. Heat and ice and massage. They probe and push and pull, gently reminding everything back into place. They ask me questions, and they listen.

Day after day I get to know the rhythm of the wellness centre they own. Day after day I watch people come in scared and hurting, and leave with information and relief. Day after day after day, until finally it starts to feel different. Until I can take a little more pressure on my shoulders, a little more weight in my messenger bag. Until it becomes clear I will never again pay rent with lifting and carrying and cleaning. Until I begin to notice the quiet chaos of their front desk, their harried looks as they treat patients and deal with insurance companies and fight with the fax machine. Until I realize I can make a difference by meeting a need.

Now, I spend my days behind that counter, answering every question and finding everything for everyone. Just the lineage I thought I wanted to avoid. Just perfect for me.

Every day I help people find their way. Find their solutions. Find their antidotes to the medical system that sees them as a disease or a discomfort. Our centre is open to everyone, but we are known for being queer/trans competent as well as welcoming. All of our providers work hard to stay informed, our naturopath the go-to doctor in our city for all things related to trans health. Overbooked and overworked, she constantly tries to fit in one more patient, one more call to an insurance company, one more consultation with a specialist, one more training of another student doctor—determined to change the experience of medicine for her patients.

The person on the other side of the counter often arrives in pain, or under duress, or rightfully angry at all the ways they have been failed and foiled in their attempts to survive. My job is to listen. To provide paperwork and answers and appointments, yes, but mostly, to listen. Sometimes they don't yet believe it's genuine, and choose to wait in the smaller lobby, away from any conversation. More often, they are so surprised to not be shut down that they can't stop talking. I listen to their histories, their frustrations and their life stories, writing none of it down. I ask what their names are, and assure them that I mean their own names, not the ones that Authority demands for paperwork. I open my eyes and heart as wide as I can, and I listen.

I understand, finally, why the women in my family did this work that pays not enough and asks for too much. Why they kept showing up to a job that rarely let them show off. They offered their tenderness as a buffer, their knowledge as an ally, and circumvented the system as often as they upheld it. Medicine alone won't suffice. Healing requires love. The providers I work with understand this. They use their hands gently, deeply, probing for ease, not faults. They push themselves to learn about what they will never live in their own bodies so as to not compound the errors and terrors already endured. They apologize when they get it wrong. They work to make it right. They listen.

WAITING ON INFORMATION FROM DOCTORS

Esther McPhee

You keep the phone nearby, read over requisition forms
at the kitchen table, steal an hour
outside, where the world smells like rosemary

and damp cedar, lit up green with rain,
until your body sends you to bed again.
Out of breath as if the wind went right through you

the way it shakes the last gold leaves pinned
against a cloudy spread of grey. You roll over
and over on the bedspread, turn the sun

on in a flicker of yellow through the window,
then off. Whole weeks pass
by you like you're in a time-lapse,

every frame captures you in a different sprawl,
now curled under a blanket, now with a book
propped against your knees, now tapping out a nonsense

rhythm on the wall. Except it all happens
in real time until you're bored out of your mind
and your body says, *Exactly.*

Get out of your mind. It doesn't care that you can't
go to work. Your body's occupied
with its own work, translating

microbial movement into pain. Which is a language
you should have studied better when you were younger
because you don't understand now

what your body's trying to tell you.
Your body doesn't understand money—if it did,
it would sure as hell expect to get paid

for all this sweat and drudgery. Your body
doesn't know how to count, not like you do,
five days wasted on sleep and movies and bad songs

on repeat. Then ten days, twenty, thirty,
then it's better to stop counting
like your body said to in the first place.

At least it never says, *I told you so.*
Your body's not worried even if you are.
It's satisfied with the snatch of blue

sky that appears through the glass
late in the afternoon, wants only to be well
enough to go touch the tangle of nasturtiums

still growing strong in the garden. Your body
puts up with your obsession with what the doctors
might tell you, even if it can't puzzle out

why you need all these words anyway.
How many times around will it take for you to realize
they don't have information for you,

not the kind you want, not the kind that gives you back
what you think you've lost. Your body
hasn't lost anything, is still a blazing

alchemy of heat and breath, still eager
to see every new sunset through your bedroom window,
that patch of sky polished to a gleam.

ACKNOWLEDGMENTS

Thank you to the Musqueam, Sḵwx̱wú7mesh, and Tsleil-Waututh peoples. As a small gesture of gratitude for living and writing on your unceded lands, I'm donating half of my royalties for *The Remedy* to Indigenous-led organizations.[1] Health is inextricably intertwined with ending, making reparations for, and healing from colonial violence. There will be no remedy without reconciliation.

Editing an anthology is one part community-building process, one part conversation, and one part puzzle assembling. It's fundamentally a labour of love—nobody's in this for the money, we're in it because we believe passionately that queer and trans stories must be told and read and shared. All of the contributors in these pages gave generously of their time, their work, and their creativity to tell their stories in *The Remedy*, so my first and biggest thank you is to them. This book wouldn't exist without you.

I'm grateful to all of the people, programs, and projects featured in our innovation profiles: Ranjith Kulatilake of Access Alliance's LGBTQ+ Newcomer Initiatives, Carly Boyce of the Affirmations Deck, Fin Gareau and Marria Townsend of the Catherine White Holman Wellness Centre, Genya Shimkin of the Q Card Project, and Kale Edmiston and Lauren Mitchell of the Trans Buddy Program. Thank you for all of the work you do—it's changing lives and creating new possibilities in queer and trans health care.

Artist and graphic facilitator Sam Bradd generously drew the illustrations that accompany these profiles. Sam's superpower is his capacity to

1 Since I hope that *The Remedy* will have a lifespan of many years, I'm committed to doing this on an ongoing basis. Thank you to Vivek Shraya for inspiring me with your actions and leadership through a similar gesture in your (extremely brilliant) poetry book, *even this page is white*.

translate words into meaningful images grounded in a deep commitment to social justice. Thank you.

Literary geniuses (and beloved friends) Amber Dawn, Ivan Coyote, and Sailor Holladay gave insightful feedback on the project and the manuscript throughout the process of creating *The Remedy*. Claire Matthews' editorial acumen helped the book shine. Leah Henderson saved the day (and my inbox) with her queer femme virgo magic.

I'm proud and grateful to again have the opportunity to work with Arsenal Pulp Press, queer cultural force and publisher of world-changing books. Special thanks to Brian Lam for his creative and editorial insights, to Oliver McPartlin for designing the beautiful cover art, and to Cynara Geissler, publicist extraordinaire (and wearer of excellent outfits).

Like everything meaningful in my life, this project wouldn't exist without the community that surrounds, sustains, and teaches me. Thank you to all of the friends who shared their ideas and health stories with me, who cheered me on throughout the process of creating this book, who helped me move (repeatedly), who made me dinner, made me laugh, made me cry, made me think, who made magic with me and reminded me that this is sacred work. I love you with all of my heart. Special thanks and extra big love to my chosen femme-ily: Amber Dawn, Eli Manning, Gisele da Silva, Rachel Rees, and Sharon Milewski. My life wouldn't be the same without you.

—Zena Sharman

INDEX

CONTRIBUTOR
BIOGRAPHIES

Lisa Baird is a writer, performance poet, facilitator, community acupuncturist, and queer white femme settler living on Attawandaron/Attawandaronk/Neutral territory (Guelph, Ontario). Her work appears or is forthcoming in *Rattle, Winter Tangerine Review, Arc Poetry Magazine, Poetry Is Dead, The Peak, The Dominion,* and elsewhere. She prefers fireflies to fireworks and would happily wear legwarmers year-round. Visit her online at lisabaird.ca.

Craig Barron's short fiction has appeared in *Glitterwolf, Chelsea Station, Event, Front&Centre, Lichen, The Air Between Us,* and *The Church-Wellesley Review.* His play, *Men Like Trees,* was presented in the Cultural Program at the 2006 International AIDS Conference. Non-fiction publications include *Xtra* and *The Globe and Mail.* Craig now writes and edits for the Community-Based Research Centre for Gay Men's Health (CBRC) in Vancouver.

Cooper Lee Bombardier is a writer and visual artist based in Portland, Oregon. His work appears in many publications and anthologies, most recently in *CutBank, Nailed Magazine, Original Plumbing,* and is forthcoming in *The Kenyon Review.* He teaches writing at Portland State University, the University of Portland, at Grant High School through Writers in The Schools, and online at LitReactor. Learn more at cooperbombardier.com.

Sam Bradd is a graphic facilitator and the principal of Drawing Change. Sam listens and draws so groups can see connections, solve problems, and lead. He's collaborated with the World Health Organization, Google, indigenous organizations, and researchers on three continents. Sam brings fifteen years of facilitation experience, a Masters in Education, and passion about visual thinking to his work. He co-edits books with the Graphic History Collective because how we tell histories can change the world.

Fayza Bundalli is a femme, South Asian writer. She is a somatic therapist, and often works at the intersections of chronic illness and disability, intergenerational trauma and resilience, and spirit. Fayza is a teacher-in-training with *generative somatics* and was an artist-in-residence with *Sins Invalid*. She is very much a Scorpio.

Cassia Chambers-Gammill is a writer and single parent living in Portland, OR. More of her essays can be found online at pdxxcollective. com. She is at work on her first poetry chapbook with a poem forthcoming in *Nimrod International Journal*.

Sand C. Chang, PhD, is a Chinese American genderqueer psychologist and trainer. They split their time between private practice and working at Kaiser Permanente's Northern California transgender clinic. Sand specializes in gender, sexuality, EMDR, addictions, and healing work with marginalized communities. Sand recently served as Chair of the APA Committee on Sexual Orientation and Gender Diversity and APA's Task Force in writing Guidelines for Psychological Practice with Transgender and Gender Nonconforming People.

Sossity Chiricuzio is a queer femme outlaw poet, a working-class radical storyteller, what her friends' parents often referred to as a bad influence, and possibly still do. A 2015 Lambda Literary Fellow, she is currently working on several projects including a hybrid memoir and is a contributing columnist at PQMonthly.com. Recent publications that include her work are *Adrienne, Glitterwolf, NANO Fiction, MashStories.com, Vine Leaves, Atlas and Alice, Wilde,* and *Glitter & Grit.* Find her online at @sossitywrites.

Caitlin Crawshaw is an award-winning essayist and freelance journalist and a recent graduate of the University of British Columbia's optional-residency creative writing MFA program. Her work has appeared in dozens of newspapers and magazines across North America, including the *Globe and Mail, Maclean's,* and *Reader's Digest.* She lives in Edmonton, Alberta, with her three-year-old daughter.

Amber Dawn is a writer, filmmaker, and performance artist, and the author of the Lambda Literary Award-winning novel *Sub Rosa,* the memoir *How Poetry Saved My Life* (winner of the Vancouver Book Award), and the poetry book *Where the words end and my body begins.* She is also editor of *Fist of the Spider Woman: Tales of Fear and Queer Desire* and co-editor of *With a Rough Tongue: Femmes Write Porn.* She has an MFA in Creative Writing (UBC), and her award-winning docuporn *Girl on Girl* has been screened in eight countries. Amber Dawn was the 2012 winner of the Writers' Trust of Canada's Dayne Ogilvie Prize for LGBT writers.

Kelli Dunham (kellidunham.com) is the ex-nun genderqueer nurse nerd comic so common in modern Brooklyn and the author of seven books including *Freak of Nurture* (Topside Press, 2014), a collection of comically tragic essays, and four young-adult health books (strangely) being used in conservative Christian homeschooling curriculum. She likes to talk about medical self advocacy, gender, and storytelling, mostly all at the same time.

Kristen L. Eckstrand, MD, PhD, is a resident psychiatrist at the University of Pittsburgh Medical Center, founder of the Vanderbilt Program for LGBT Health, Chair of the Association of American Medical Colleges' Advisory Committee on Sexual Orientation, Gender Identity, and Sex Development, and Vice President for Education of GLMA: Health Professionals Advancing LGBT Equality. She is committed to advancing health equity and improving health care for LGBT individuals through research, clinical practice, and health professions education.

Eli Erlick is a queer trans woman, activist, and director of Trans Student Educational Resources. Her work and writing focus on trans and queer organizations, youth, education, linguistics, identities, media, and health. Her work can be found on her website at elierlick.com.

Ariel Estrella, who hails from Queens, NY, is a queer Latinx advocate focused on fostering beloved communities. They recently graduated with a B.A. from Macalester College as a Mellon Mays Undergraduate Fellow. For three years, they wrote a column for their college newspaper, "The Mac Weekly," on intimate health, surviving violence, and the politics of love. They currently work at a social justice arts organization with plans of returning to academia soon.

Sailor Holladay is a writer, teacher, textile artist, and asset developer for low-income communities in Oregon. Sailor was a Lambda Literary Fellow in 2012 and holds an MFA in Creative Nonfiction from Mills College. Sailor is proud to have been off drugs since 2005. Find out more at sailorholladay.com.

Francisco Ibàñez-Carrasco, PhD (1999, Simon Fraser University) came to Canada from Chile in 1985 and has lived and loved with HIV since. He is a lifelong educationist with current focus on eLearning, a creative non-fiction writer (givingitraw.ca), and a health scientist in HIV with focus on ageing, sexuality and rehabilitation. He lives in Toronto with his husband and his fat cat Orion.

Xeph Kalma is a trans woman of colour surviving in Toronto. She loves love and to be loved, and has a particular affinity for creatures with four legs. She also enjoys justice.

Keiko Lane is a Japanese American poet, essayist, and psychotherapist writing about the intersections of queer culture, oppression resistance, racial and gender justice, HIV criminalization, and reproductive justice. Her current writing projects focus on queer kinship and queer rage and grief in long-term survivors of ACT UP and Queer Nation. A psychotherapist in Berkeley, CA, she also teaches graduate psychotherapy courses on queer and multicultural psychotherapies, the psychodynamics of social justice, and the embodied literature of exile.

Esther McPhee is a writer, magic-maker, and collective organizer who grew up on Stó:lō land and now lives on Musqueam, Squamish, and Tsleil-Waututh land in Vancouver, where they earned an MFA in Creative Writing from UBC. Their writing has appeared across North America. Esther likes poetry, pop music, and scavenging for berries. They're one-half of the organizing team behind REVERB: A Queer Reading Series and can be visited online at esthermcphee.com.

A. K. Morrissey got involved with this book project as an independent scholar. Morrissey's primary form of writing recently has been papers that have been selected for presentation at a variety of academic conferences across North America. Some of the common foci throughout Morrissey's work include space, concepts of power, intersectionality, assemblage, privilege/marginalization, asexuality, nonlibidinal experience, trans/gender-variance, disability, queerness, and feminism.

soma navidson is your everyday subversive queer. She is a blogger, poet, workshop facilitator, dressmaker, and all-around crafty radical who also studies and works in health care. soma's work is rooted in harm reduction and primarily revolves around housing justice, prison abolition, queer and trans liberation, and fighting the drug war. Some of her thoughts on nursing and the medical industrial complex can be found at her blog: nursingroar.tumblr.com.

Rita O'Link is a Community Relations Representative for TgInnerselves, the Sudbury-based transgender support group, and also volunteers with a number of other organizations. Rita has had a lifelong struggle with being transgender, and is working hard to try and help those in her family deal with her transition. This chapter of her life has yet to be written.

Ahmed Danny Ramadan is an experienced journalist with bylines appearing in the *Washington Post*, *The Guardian*, and *Foreign Policy*. Currently Danny is the Volunteer Coordinator at QMUNITY—BC's Queer Resource Centre. An author with two collections of short stories published in Arabic, he is planning to publish his first novel in English soon. A jack-of-all-trades who found his calling in activism, civil society, journalism, and creative writing as well as his personal experience as a former gay refugee; Danny is passionate about the values of volunteerism and democracy, and the causes of social justice and LGBTQ refugees' rights.

Margaret Robinson is a feminist scholar from Nova Scotia and a member of the Lennox Island First Nation. Her work examines mental health and substance use in Indigenous and Settler populations, especially among sexual and gender minority people. She is currently a Researcher in Residence in Indigenous Health at the Ontario HIV Treatment Network and an Affiliate Research Scientist at the Centre for Addiction & Mental Health in Toronto.

Sinclair Sexsmith is a genderqueer kinky butch writer who teaches and performs, specializing in sexualities, genders, and relationships. They've written at sugarbutch.net since 2006, which is recognized by numerous places as one of the Top Sex Blogs. Sinclair's gender theory and queer erotica is widely published online and in more than twenty anthologies; they edited *Best Lesbian Erotica 2012* and *Say Please: Lesbian BDSM Erotica*, and authored *Sweet & Rough: Queer Kink Erotica*. Sinclair uses the pronouns they/them/theirs/themself.

Vivek Shraya is a Toronto-based artist whose body of work includes several albums, films, and books, which have been used as textbooks at several post-secondary institutions. Her debut novel, *She of the Mountains*, was named one of *The Globe and Mail*'s Best Books of 2014. Vivek is a three-time Lambda Literary Award finalist, a 2015 Toronto Arts Foundation Emerging Artist Award finalist, and a 2015 recipient of the Writers' Trust of Canada's Dayne Ogilvie Prize Honour of Distinction.

Kara Sievewright is a queer writer, artist, and designer who mainly creates comics. She has published comics, writing, and illustrations in many magazines and anthologies including *Plenitude, Drawn to Change: Graphic Histories of Working-Class Struggle, Descant, filling Station*, and *Briarpatch*. She has an MFA in Creative Writing from UBC and is a member of the Graphic History Collective. She lives in Daajing Giids Llnagaay/Queen Charlotte, Haida Gwaii as a settler on Haida Territory with her partner. You can see more of her work at makerofnets.ca.

j wallace skelton is very concerned about how gender stereotypes and gendered assumptions shape and limit our experiences and possibilities, and works to create more possibilities for all of us, especially children. j works for the Gender-Based Violence Prevention office of the Toronto District School Board, studies how to create schools that are more celebratory of gender diversity at the Ontario Institute for Studies in Education (OISE) and writes about gender anywhere he can. More at juxtaposeconsulting.com and ishai-wallace.livejournal.com.

Kyle Shaughnessy is a Métis (Dene, Ukrainian, & Irish), trans, queer, husband, storyteller, and social worker who grew up in rural BC and the Northwest Territories. He currently works in the public health care system, supporting adult allies to create safer rural communities for transgender youth. Through his enthusiasm for writing, facilitating, and public speaking,

Kyle firmly believes in the power of personal narrative to connect queer and trans experiences, and to create social change.

Sean Saifa Wall is an intersex activist, collage artist, and writer. He is the founder of EMERGE (saifaemerges.com), a project that increases social impact through visual artistry. EMERGE is the compilation of his life work that is grounded in community encompassing both his activist and creative contributions. He originally hails from the Bronx, but lived in the San Francisco Bay Area before settling in Atlanta, Georgia, which he calls home for now.

Jenna J. Webber is a small-town Northern Ontarian with big dreams and a personality to match. She completed a Bachelor of Health Sciences Honours degree at McMaster University before attending the Northern Ontario School of Medicine MD program, from which she is scheduled to graduate in 2017. She is the 2015/2016 National Officer of Reproductive and Sexual Health with the Canadian Federation of Medical Students and is passionate about LGBTQ+ health, advocacy, and wellness.

Chase Willier is Nehiyaw from Saddle Lake Cree Nation and Sucker Creek First Nation in Alberta. He was part of the Sixties Scoop and grew up in the Syilx Nation where he was traditionally adopted. Chase spent thirty years in the RCMP working with First Nations as a two spirit woman before he retired and transitioned. He is presently writing his memoir and is happily married with a new baby girl.

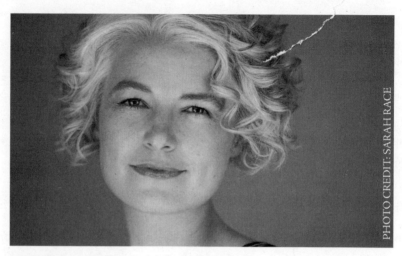

Zena Sharman is a femme force of nature and a passionate advocate for queer and trans health. She has over a decade's experience in health research, including seven years as the Assistant Director of Canada's national gender and health research funding institute. Zena co-chairs the board of the Catherine White Holman Wellness Centre, a holistic health care centre for transgender and gender-diverse communities. She served on the board of the Canadian Professional Association for Transgender Health from 2013 to 2015.

Zena co-edited the Lambda Literary Award-nominated anthology *Persistence: All Ways Butch and Femme* (Arsenal Pulp Press, 2011), and she's presented on gender, sexuality, and health to audiences across North America. *The Remedy* brings together her love of writing and stories with her commitment to making the world a healthier and more equitable place. Zena has a PhD in Interdisciplinary Studies from the University of British Columbia. Her resume also includes party thrower, cabaret host, go-go dancer for a queer punk band, campus radio DJ, and elementary school public speaking champion. She lives in Vancouver.